C000011091

HEALTHY EATING FOR LIFE

Healthy Eating for LIFE

An Intuitive Eating Workbook to Stop Dieting Forever

CARA HARBSTREET, MS, RD, LD

ALTHEA
PRESS

TO ANYONE WHO SEEKS FOOD FREEDOM IN A CULTURE
THAT WORKS SO HARD TO TAKE IT AWAY FROM THEM.

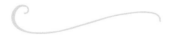

Copyright © 2019 by Althea Press, Emeryville, California

No part of this publication may be reproduced, stored in a retrieval system, or transmitted in any form or by any means, electronic, mechanical, photocopying, recording, scanning, or otherwise, except as permitted under Sections 107 or 108 of the 1976 United States Copyright Act, without the prior written permission of the Publisher. Requests to the Publisher for permission should be addressed to the Permissions Department, Althea Press, 6005 Shellmound Street, Suite 175, Emeryville, CA 94608.

Limit of Liability/Disclaimer of Warranty: The Publisher and the author make no representations or warranties with respect to the accuracy or completeness of the contents of this work and specifically disclaim all warranties, including without limitation warranties of fitness for a particular purpose. No warranty may be created or extended by sales or promotional materials. The advice and strategies contained herein may not be suitable for every situation. This work is sold with the understanding that the Publisher is not engaged in rendering medical, legal, or other professional advice or services. If professional assistance is required, the services of a competent professional person should be sought. Neither the Publisher nor the author shall be liable for damages arising herefrom. The fact that an individual, organization, or website is referred to in this work as a citation and/or potential source of further information does not mean that the author or the Publisher endorses the information the individual, organization, or website may provide or recommendations they/it may make. Further, readers should be aware that websites listed in this work may have changed or disappeared between when this work was written and when it is read.

For general information on our other products and services or to obtain technical support, please contact our Customer Care Department within the United States at (866) 744-2665, or outside the United States at (510) 253-0500.

Althea Press publishes its books in a variety of electronic and print formats. Some content that appears in print may not be available in electronic books, and vice versa.

TRADEMARKS: Althea Press and the Althea Press logo are trademarks or registered trademarks of Callisto Media Inc. and/or its affiliates, in the United States and other countries, and may not be used without written permission. All other trademarks are the property of their respective owners. Althea Press is not associated with any product or vendor mentioned in this book.

Interior and Cover Designer: William Mack
Editor: Lauren Ladoceour
Production Editor: Erum Khan

ISBN: Print 978-1-64152-490-2 | eBook 978-1-64152-491-9

CONTENTS

Introduction: The Non-Diet Difference vi

Chapter One
Eating Intuitively 1

Chapter Two
Break Out of the
Diet Trap 20

Chapter Three
Listen to Your Body 38

Chapter Four
Feed Your Hunger 57

Chapter Five
Healthy Food,
Healthy Choices 76

Chapter Six
Change for Life 99

Resources 112

References 115

Index 120

THE NON-DIET DIFFERENCE

WHEN I FIRST BECAME A DIETITIAN, I fully bought into the idea that health could be improved through dieting. Dieting was so common that I thought it was both normal and appropriate. At the same time, I was struggling with my own issues: problematic fear and suspicion of food, compulsive exercise habits, and deep shame about my body and appearance. If you're holding this book, you or someone you care about has likely been in those same shoes. Maybe you have felt beholden to a label you've placed on your food habits, helpless to break the cycle of emotional eating, or unable to step away from rigid meal prep and planning. Intuitive eating can change this mentality for you, just as it has for me and many of my clients.

Intuitive eating is *not* a diet. It is 180-degree pivot from traditional diets. It makes you the expert of your body. You learn to trust foods that were previously off-limits or made you feel out of control. Cravings are honored instead of repressed. And you grant yourself the freedom to eat what and how much you want while reconnecting with natural cues for when to start and stop eating.

By simply becoming curious about intuitive eating, you're taking a big step toward creating a healthier relationship with food and your body. Chances are you've already invested in other books, programs, coaches—you name it—in the pursuit of changing the way you eat. But no matter how or why you arrived here, I want you to know it is possible to free yourself from restrictions, prescriptive exercise routines, meal plans, and diets masquerading as frustrating "lifestyles." This book places the power back in your hands. As you work through the chapters and exercises, you'll find:

- Habit-formation strategies that are sustainable
- Basic psychological tools to support positive behavior change

- Opportunities to reflect on and become attuned to your body, what you need, and what you want
- A compassionate, adaptable, evidence-based approach to well-being

A great irony hit me during my own efforts to heal my relationship with food through intuitive eating. When I started out, it seemed all I could do was think about food. I was more aware than ever of the sheer number of meal-related decisions I made every day. Decision fatigue is real and exhausting, and I often questioned whether intuitive eating was worth it.

As a few weeks passed, though, I realized I was spending less time overthinking every little bite that went into my mouth. Eventually, making decisions about food became second nature; I could plan or sit down for a meal without thoughts of food consuming every moment of the experience. Whatever I'd put on my plate wasn't "good" or "bad." It was neutral. The practices truly started to feel intuitive, and that progress freed up so much mental space and energy. Liberating? Yes. Empowering? Definitely. The effort to get to that point had been worth it.

Don't be discouraged by the initial effort of your new way of eating. Intuitive eating is anything but easy in the beginning. Patience and persistence are key to unlearning diet culture's food rules and replacing those rules with your own wisdom about your body and values. That's why I recommend reading this workbook from start to finish rather than skipping around. Work through it slowly—don't try to finish it in a single session. Take it one chapter and one tool at a time, letting each practice sink in before proceeding. Even if it's only for a few moments each day, try to set some time aside to reflect, journal, discuss, read, or learn.

You'll start by learning what it means to eat intuitively and how to identify any sneaky, lingering diet habits. You'll see the impact that restriction has on your mind and body, and you'll develop compassion for yourself instead of judgment. Then, you'll focus on listening to what your body truly needs with practices to help you reconnect with sensations of hunger and fullness. You'll also learn what it means to eat mindfully. Then, you'll take back your power by examining the mind-body connection and getting to the root of your cravings.

When you're ready, nutrition will come back into the equation and you'll begin building balanced meals and snacks you truly enjoy. You'll look at what being active does for you when a better physique isn't the goal. And, in the final chapter, you'll take stock of your victories (and challenges) to see how to use all your new tools and practices to pave a new path forward. You will have plenty of time to complete the exercises, and you may find it helpful to repeat or revisit them. Questions posed throughout this workbook will give you additional opportunities to journal.

The path to intuitive eating is not linear, so be prepared for challenges, triggers, or setbacks. Rather than approach intuitive eating as a goal to cross off a checklist, think of it as your opportunity to focus on yourself for a few moments every day. Intuitive eating is a small gift to yourself, an act of self-care that will benefit you in the long run.

CHAPTER ONE

EATING

Intuitively

YOU'VE BEEN TAUGHT that to be healthy, you need to eat a certain way or adhere to a lifestyle that epitomizes good health. That might mean counting calories, tracking macros, measuring food, prepping days' worth of meals, or following a strict exercise program. With intuitive eating, there are no food rules or rigid meal plans. If those rules or plans are what you're accustomed to seeking, you're not alone. The diet industry is a $60 billion juggernaut for a reason. It's normal and valid to desire what it promises to provide, be it feeling more comfortable in your own skin, having the energy to play with your children, or fitting into anything in your closet.

Even if you haven't been "on a diet," you've likely adopted some of its behaviors—like vilifying certain foods—or experienced restrictive thoughts. The truth is, restriction often only makes the things you're avoiding more tempting. It's like trying to tell yourself not to think about the color blue. The moment you say "don't" or "I can't," your mind immediately focuses on that exact thing, deflecting attention from your body's needs and cues about when, what, and how much to eat.

The Benefits of Intuitive Eating

Studies have shown that the way to break free of unhealthy eating habits (and otherwise not fall off the wagon) is not to return to restriction; it's to give yourself permission, which is a large part of learning to eat intuitively. There are many benefits to flipping the restriction script, including:

ENDING THE FOOD FIGHT. If food is no longer the enemy, you are free to enjoy the experience of eating, whether it's a solo mindful meal or a boisterous social event.

CHANGING THE RANKS. If you're able to look at ingredients and meals in a neutral way, gone is their power to control you. Instead, they're there to support and serve you—not the other way around.

RECONNECTING WITH YOUR BODY. No more questioning your hunger or fullness. You can trust what your body is trying to tell you and move confidently through the day with more peace of mind about food-related decisions.

MINIMIZING CHAOS. Becoming an intuitive eater means you'll benefit from the freedom of a non-diet approach and have opportunities to build a flexible structure that promotes good self-care.

DISCOVERING A HOLISTIC APPROACH TO WELL-BEING. "Health" is much more than regular visits to the doctor, adequate sleep, and "clean" living. Without a fixation on food, you'll have space to consider your needs in the areas of emotional, mental, social, financial, and spiritual health.

Getting Started

The beauty of intuitive eating is that there's no "right" or "wrong" way to begin. It's enough to simply become more curious about why and how you're eating. This practice looks different for everyone, and the amount of time you need to devote to it may depend on the length and intensity of your past struggles. Likewise, certain situations—like traveling or the holidays—might prompt you to focus more on these skills than when you're settled in a "normal" routine. Diets offer time-bound guarantees; intuitive eating equips you with tools that make dieting unnecessary. It's a commitment to reject your old habits for good, so allow it to take the time it takes, and keep a notebook handy for journaling prompts and short exercises along the way.

Rest assured, there will come a moment for turning your attention to what you're eating. But for now, let's reflect on how you feel toward food, exercise, and health. Doing so can crack open the door and build confidence as you enter this world of eating more intuitively.

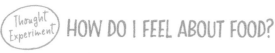 HOW DO I FEEL ABOUT FOOD?

Ask yourself how often you engage in the following behaviors. Afterward, if you see that you mostly checked off "Always" or "Often," you may already be practicing intuitive eating to some degree. If you notice you marked "Rarely" or "Never" more often than not, a dieting mentality may be driving a lot of your decisions or thoughts about food. Either way, this book is for you. Feel free to return to this exercise anytime you want to see how you've changed your eating habits.

I trust that my body can handle an unusually large meal, and eating past my fullness does not bother me much.

☑ ALWAYS ☐ OFTEN ☐ SOMETIMES ☐ RARELY ☐ NEVER

I eat a wide variety of food.

☐ ALWAYS ☑ OFTEN ☐ SOMETIMES ☐ RARELY ☐ NEVER

I include foods that some might consider high in sugar, fat, or calories.

☐ ALWAYS ☐ OFTEN ☑ SOMETIMES ☐ RARELY ☐ NEVER

I can easily sense my hunger or fullness based on how my body feels.

☐ ALWAYS ☐ OFTEN ☐ SOMETIMES ☐ RARELY ☑ NEVER

I can take a rest day or break from exercise without feeling anxious.

☐ ALWAYS ☐ OFTEN ☑ SOMETIMES ☐ RARELY ☐ NEVER

If I eat for emotional reasons, it does not impact how I eat or if I eat more afterward.

☐ ALWAYS ☐ OFTEN ☐ SOMETIMES ☐ RARELY ☑ NEVER

I have a self-care routine that includes ways to take care of my mental, emotional, and physical health.

☐ ALWAYS ☑ OFTEN ☐ SOMETIMES ☐ RARELY ☐ NEVER

I avoid labeling foods as "good" or "bad."

☐ ALWAYS ☐ OFTEN ☑ SOMETIMES ☐ RARELY ☐ NEVER

I move my body because I enjoy the way it makes me feel.

☐ ALWAYS   ☑ OFTEN   ☐ SOMETIMES   ☐ RARELY   ☐ NEVER

When I exercise, I don't think about how many calories I'm burning or what it could make my body look like.

☐ ALWAYS   ☐ OFTEN   ☐ SOMETIMES   ☑ RARELY   ☐ NEVER

Comments from friends or family about what I'm eating do not usually bother me.

☐ ALWAYS   ☐ OFTEN   ☑ SOMETIMES   ☐ RARELY   ☐ NEVER

Comments from strangers about what I'm eating do not usually bother me.

☑ ALWAYS   ☐ OFTEN   ☐ SOMETIMES   ☐ RARELY   ☐ NEVER

Comments from friends or family about my weight do not usually bother me.

☑ ALWAYS   ☐ OFTEN   ☐ SOMETIMES   ☐ RARELY   ☑ NEVER

Comments from strangers about my weight do not usually bother me.

☑ ALWAYS   ☐ OFTEN   ☐ SOMETIMES   ☐ RARELY   ☐ NEVER

I feel comfortable asking for my food boundaries to be respected.

☐ ALWAYS   ☐ OFTEN   ☑ SOMETIMES   ☐ RARELY   ☐ NEVER

I base my food choices on what I want.

☐ ALWAYS   ☐ OFTEN   ☑ SOMETIMES   ☐ RARELY   ☐ NEVER

I base my food choices on what I know will fill me up and satisfy me.

☐ ALWAYS   ☐ OFTEN   ☑ SOMETIMES   ☐ RARELY   ☐ NEVER

I feel confident ordering food at restaurants even if I don't see the menu in advance.

☐ ALWAYS   ☐ OFTEN   ☐ SOMETIMES   ☑ RARELY   ☐ NEVER

I have opportunities to practice mindful eating.

☐ ALWAYS   ☐ OFTEN   ☐ SOMETIMES   ☑ RARELY   ☐ NEVER

It's not a problem for me if I sometimes have distractions while I eat.

☐ ALWAYS   ☐ OFTEN   ☑ SOMETIMES   ☐ RARELY   ☐ NEVER

Meal planning is helpful, not stressful.

☐ ALWAYS   ☐ OFTEN   ☐ SOMETIMES   ☑ RARELY   ☐ NEVER

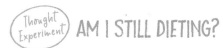

AM I STILL DIETING?

Even if you're not doing the newest fad diet or following a strict set of rules, you may be dieting in other ways. Restriction isn't just the physical act of eating less food; it's also your thoughts and attitudes toward what you allow yourself to have and enjoy. Consider whether you're doing any of the following things and whether you're ready to start letting them go to become a more intuitive eater. Add to this list as you become more aware of the subtle ways that dieting lingers in your life. The work you're doing with this book will help you shed these habits and prove how they're no longer serving you.

- Counting calories, points, or servings so you don't eat too much
- Weighing or counting food portions to avoid eating too much
- Avoiding certain foods if you feel they have too many calories, points, or grams
- Basing your food choices at a restaurant or party on nutritional data, not whether you want it
- Always choosing "diet" or "nonfat" versions of drinks and foods
- Weighing yourself often or multiple times per day
- Choosing exercise based on how many calories you think you'll burn or to make up for something you ate
- Classifying foods based on their nutrition content, or labeling them as "good" or "bad," "clean" or "dirty," "sinful" or "guilt-free"
- Using a label like "vegetarian/vegan" or "gluten-free" or "whole food" or "clean eating" to disguise or hide your desire to control how much you eat, rather than cultivating your true food or lifestyle preference
- Associating your eating habits with your personal identity
- Feeling anxiety or stress at a meal if you don't know how many calories it has

- Periodically detoxing, fasting, eating less and/or exercising more for an upcoming event or to "get back on track"

- _____

- _____

- _____

- _____

Changes for the Better

How much time have you spent wishing, hoping, and worrying about things that are beyond your control? You're not alone. Intuitive eating helps you let go of what you can't change and encourages you to focus on behaviors that can positively impact your health and well-being. Here are some examples of what you do have the power to control:

- Eating in a way that nourishes and satisfies you
- Engaging in forms of movement that you enjoy
- Getting adequate sleep
- Practicing self-care
- Supporting your mental health and cultivating healthy relationships
- Avoiding risky behavior
- Seeking preventative health care and/or managing a condition

JOURNAL: _Take some time to reflect on where some of your current beliefs about food, health, or your body originated. What would you add to the previous list? Do you still believe them to be true, or can you recognize them as false beliefs that you can start to let go of?_

To fully embrace intuitive eating and make positive changes, it's helpful to first examine some of your most deeply held beliefs about food, health, and your body. It's easy to confuse your personal values with what society values, though occasionally the two can align. But more often than not, the stuff you think is the most important is skewed by the environment you live in. Here are some of the many examples of the external forces that influence our values:

- Your family and friends and their attitudes toward food, health, and bodies
- Magazines, social media, movies, celebrity culture

- Traditional or conventional health care settings that are weight-centric
- Social spaces, such as the office, gym, or other public places

WHAT MATTERS MOST TO YOU?

Values are not the same as goals. They're also not the same as the qualities or characteristics you want to display to the world. Think of values as the guardrails that can keep you pointed in the general direction in which you want your life to move. Goals are the things you encounter or accomplish along the way. They are time-oriented, whereas values are ongoing. Goals may be temporarily motivating; values continuously drive you forward. For example:

GOAL I want to improve my fitness.

VALUES Health, longevity

GOAL I want to feel comfortable at the pool with friends.

VALUES Acceptance, confidence, inclusion

GOAL I want to stop obsessing about eating at family gatherings.

VALUES Being present with family

The next two exercises can help you distinguish between goals and values, as well as determine what's most important to you, even if it differs from what is expected of you.

IF YOU NEED MORE SUPPORT

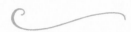

Intuitive eating may or may not be appropriate for someone recovering from a clinical eating disorder. Eating disorders are serious mental illnesses, and it's imperative to seek professional help if you're struggling with:

- Anorexia nervosa
- Bulimia nervosa
- Binge eating disorder
- Eating disorder not otherwise specified (EDNOS)
- Extreme or debilitating anxiety around food or eating, suicidal thoughts or ideation, or other efforts to self-harm

Eating disorders don't discriminate. They impact people of any age, gender or sexual identity, ethnicity, ability, education, or income level. And although not all forms of disordered eating are clinically recognized and diagnosed, anyone with disordered eating or an eating disorder deserves to heal and recover. Here are a few national resources that can support you in your step toward recovery:

National Eating Disorders Association Helpline: 800-931-2237

Eating Disorder Referral & Information Center (edreferral.com)

Families Empowered and Supporting Treatment of Eating Disorders (FEAST) (feast-ed.org)

WHAT I SAY VS. WHAT I WANT AND VALUE

What you value could be quite different than what someone else values. It's also not unusual for values to change as you move through life, so revisiting this exercise can help you see if what you prioritize today still resonates in the future. In the table that follows, you can see some examples of how what you value can be disguised by what you say. By digging further or repeatedly asking, "But why?" or "What do I really want?" you can home in on your honest-to-goodness value. Take some time to consider which of these examples resonates with you, and then add some of your own in the space provided.

WHAT I SAY	WHAT I WANT	VALUE THAT ALIGNS WITH WHAT I WANT
"I want to be thin."	To be comfortable and confident in my body	Connection, trust, compassion, acceptance,
"I shouldn't eat that."	Less guilt or shame around food	Fun, peace, ease, exploration, curiosity
"I need to change."	To be accepted and to accept myself	Growth (personal or professional), courage, boldness
"I have to follow these rules."	To be able to trust my choices	Confidence, knowledge
"I don't have enough discipline."	For things to be easier	Commitment, competence
"I'm addicted to food."	To feel like I'm in control	Health, autonomy, authenticity
"Diets don't work for me."	Something sustainable that lasts	Security, dependability, genuineness
"This is how it will always be."	Predictability, familiarity, simplicity	Tradition, loyalty

TWO SIDES OF THE SAME COIN

Select a value from the previous section that you'd like to focus on first. Perhaps it's a value that feels approachable at this point, or one from which you sense the greatest disconnect. As much as you may dislike thinking about suffering or vulnerability (especially your own), it may be that your values and suffering are two sides of the same coin. In that case, you likely care deeply about your values, which can cause you to feel vulnerable or alone; therefore, in an effort to alleviate your suffering, you may also move further away from your values. Examining this relationship between values and suffering may be uncomfortable but it is valuable.

1. Choose a piece of paper or an index card to be your two-sided coin. Name the value with which you want to start, and write it at the top. Then, list the things that will move you in the direction aligning with that particular value.

2. Flip the paper over and write "Suffering" at the top. List the potentially uncomfortable aspects of the actions you just listed—for example, unpleasant memories, highly judgmental thoughts, or deeply held fears.

3. Ask yourself: If I avoid these things that cause me to suffer, am I also willing to let go of my value? (Revisit the list you made in What I Say vs. What I Want and Value on the previous page.)

4. What might happen if you start to take those actions? What might happen if you don't?

There is no right or wrong response. This exercise is simply meant to show you what might realistically happen if you begin to align your choices and actions more closely with your values.

Health from the Inside Out

One of the reasons diets fail is that they're time-oriented and often linked to a specific outcome (typically weight loss, a smaller clothing size, or some other change to your body). This goal is shortsighted, and it also emphasizes that your value and worth are connected to your appearance and ability to change or maintain it.

Throughout this workbook, you'll be challenged to think about health differently. Of course, physical health is important for matters other than weight or appearance. But keep in mind that no one is obligated to pursue health (or the same version of health as what is expected or assumed).

WHAT DOES HEALTHY MEAN TO YOU?

"Healthy" is a tricky word to define, so take your time with this exercise to get clarity on what it really looks like for you. You might immediately think of physical health and perhaps mental or emotional health, too. But what about other dimensions of wellness? Write a few sentences about what you aspire to have in each area of your life. What would it look like for you to be truly healthy?

_____

_____

_____

PHYSICAL HEALTH How do I want to feel? What do I consider to be a high quality of life? How do I want to age? What do I want to be able to do with my body?

_____

_____

_____

MENTAL AND EMOTIONAL HEALTH What would it look like to have harmony in my life? How can I acknowledge and tend to how I'm feeling? What resources can help me do that?

_____

_____

_____

FINANCIAL HEALTH How would my financial situation look different if I changed my eating or health habits? What could I do with that money instead? Are there other areas of my health or well-being in which I'd like to invest?

_____

_____

_____

SPIRITUAL HEALTH What is my purpose or calling in life? Can I form a deeper connection with my faith or explore different ways to fulfill myself?

_____

_____

_____

RELATIONSHIPS How am I taking care of my relationships? (This can include family, friends, colleagues, and neighbors.) What could my healthy relationships look like with the key people in my life?

_____

_____

_____

Now, look at which responses are similar to the healthy life you described at the top. Which areas could use some help aligning with what you've written?

HEALTHY EATING: MYTHS VS. FACTS TABLE

Your health is not a problem that needs to be solved, but you may have been sold that idea. There's an overwhelming amount of information available; some of it is rooted in facts, but a lot of it is simply false. Take some time to consider the table that follows, and start seeking out false beliefs. For more insight, return to the What I Say vs. What I Want and Value exercise on page 10 that helped you identify your values. Continue to challenge the beliefs you may start to recognize as being untrue.

WHAT I'VE BEEN TOLD	MYTH OR FACT?	THE TRUTH
I have to lose weight to be healthy.	Myth	Weight is not an indicator of health; health is a spectrum, and there is a full range of healthfulness in people of all shapes, sizes, ages, and abilities.
It's important that I get healthy.	Myth	Health is not a moral obligation that you owe to anyone. If this is something you value, it may be important to you, but whether or not you choose to pursue good health is a personal choice.
Intuitive eating means I just eat when I'm hungry and stop when I'm full.	Somewhat of a fact—but there's so much more to it than that.	This is a sneaky form of dieting, also called the hunger-fullness diet. It's a form of careful or restrained eating, and although intuitive eating includes some focus on hunger, appetite, and satiety, this is an overly simplified version.
Emotional eating is always a negative thing.	Myth	Emotional eating is one coping mechanism and may be problematic if it's your only coping mechanism. But people eat for a number of reasons and emotions, including happy ones.

WHAT I'VE BEEN TOLD	MYTH OR FACT?	THE TRUTH
I have no self-control or discipline around food	Myth	It might ring true, but it's not. While it's possible to feel addicted to or controlled by food, this is often the side effect of restriction. Self-control (or lack thereof) is not the reason why some people remain thin or why some people fail to lose weight.
A new, trendy food program I just read about is a lifestyle, not a diet.	Myth	If the goal is to make some bodies smaller or it has a focus on appearance over health or happiness, it's still a diet.
Healthy eating looks the same for everyone.	Myth	Food is highly personal. What's healthy for someone can be a deadly allergen to someone else, so "healthy" is a relative term. It can look drastically different from person to person, and even different for the same person day to day or week to week.

WHAT'S A HABIT ANYWAY?

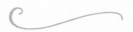

There's some debate when it comes to defining a habit. However, researchers tend to agree that to be considered a habit, an action must:

1. Occur regularly
2. Be triggered by a situation or something in your environment
3. Occur without much or any thought

Consider habits that get triggered by day-to-day events. There are always fascinating and insightful patterns to draw from what you notice. Take your observations one step further and think about the consequences of your habits. With time and repetition, new habits can replace old ones as you relearn what it means to trust your body. Eventually, making informed and empowered decisions about food will become intuitive.

After all, intuitive eating is a self-guided process. You and you alone are the foremost expert of your body and what you experience while living in it. The habits you choose to focus on will be determined by whether or not you prefer to make a change in how you respond to a trigger.

Much of the conversation about building habits revolves around how you respond to a cue or trigger in your environment. What if you could form a new habit by *removing* a cue or trigger? What would your habits look like if you deleted a tracking app from your phone? Or unfollowed social media accounts that made you feel inadequate? What if you stopped surrounding yourself with people who bash their bodies or use food-shaming language? It's tough to challenge old habits, but you may be surprised by the new ones that form when diet culture is removed from your environment.

It may take weeks, months, even years to build or rebuild the habits most important to you. Subsequent sections of this workbook will invite you to create a new habit around one aspect of intuitive eating. Perhaps one of the most difficult aspects of forming new habits and letting go of old ones is forging a new identity. Transitioning away from dieting or a certain style of eating may mean grappling with the idea that you are no longer a "dieter" or some other self-identifying label. When an obstacle like this arises, remember that intuitive eating is an ongoing process. Be kind to yourself, and know that it's perfectly normal to feel a little uncomfortable while changing your identity. A new one—that only you can define for yourself—is just around the bend.

GET TO KNOW YOUR HABITS

Which of your actions are driven by your own **internal cue** (aka inner wisdom), and which are **mindless habits** or **external cues**? To tell the difference, see if you can suss out which habits and cues underlay the actions in the following list. Add to the list any actions (and the habits and cues underlaying them) that come to mind in the space provided at the end.

- Eating such a large dinner that you feel uncomfortably full because you didn't eat enough during the day, and now you're ravenous **(internal cue)**
- Pushing through a workout when your body feels sore or tired because that's what you have scheduled **(internal cue)**
- Grabbing a handful of candy from the jar on your assistant's desk when you walk in **(mindless habit)**
- Eating the samples at Costco or Sam's Club, regardless of whether or not you're hungry **(mindless habit)**
- Opening the refrigerator and grabbing a snack because you walked into the kitchen **(mindless habit)**
- Drinking water to numb your appetite because it's not time to eat yet according to your meal plan **(external cue)**
- Snacking on the ingredients you use to cook dinner as you're preparing the meal **(mindless habit)**
- Avoiding a particular food because you know it leads to GI symptoms or makes you feel less than your best **(internal cue)**

- _____

- _____

- _____

- _____

Put a star next to any actions on this list that you'd like to change in the future. Those that stem from mindless habits are not necessarily "wrong" or "bad." But becoming attuned to these actions can help you form new habits based on what you intuitively know your body needs.

Takeaways

- Intuitive eating is not a diet and will never use body weight, shape, or size as a measure of "success."

- Intuitive eating can help anyone improve or heal their relationship with food and their body, regardless of past experiences or health concerns.

- Everyone's journey with intuitive eating will look different. It's about identifying your values, not comparing yourself to others.

- You will be challenged or feel frustrated, and that's okay. Keeping a journal may be helpful to continue working on these things as they come up.

- If you are grappling with a diagnosed eating disorder or are seeking more support, please reach out to a professional trained in intuitive eating, such as a registered dietitian, certified intuitive eating counselor, therapist, or an eating disorder treatment program.

CHAPTER TWO

Break Out
of the
DIET
TRAP

IF DIET CULTURE WERE A MOVIE, it might look a lot like 2004's *Mean Girls*. The Tina Fey flick showed a high schooler's attempt to fit in by following a clique's random rules on fashion and food—among other things—all the while not flinching at the clique's silver-tongued scrutiny. Like the movie's queen bees, diet culture is a mean girl. It's the critical voice in your head shaming your meal choices, labeling them as "good" or "bad," and judging your appearance at every turn. It determines the arbitrary (and often ridiculous) food guidelines that you impose on yourself. Meanwhile, you want so desperately to fit in that you risk losing yourself in the process. You willingly trade your authentic self or go along with the crowd for the chance to be socially accepted. You may do this even when it feels wrong. You do it because that's what you know and that's what everybody around you seems to be doing.

By the time the film credits roll, each character has achieved a happy ending by overcoming their fear of judgment and letting go of the clique's expectations. In real life, relinquishing expectations and fear takes longer than 97 minutes. To make peace with your body and food, you have to reject the idea that dieting is the only way to fit in. That "mean girl" voice in your mind is standing between you and a practice that supports how you want to live.

Diets and the Culture of No

Imagine hearing a commercial for a new wellness procedure. It's only effective for about 5 percent of the people who use it. The other 95 percent may experience temporary success but then feel even worse than they did before. Nearly everyone reports some kind of physical or psychological side effect, even though the procedure is highly recommended. Satisfaction levels are low, mental health suffers, and small fortunes are spent.

Does that sound like a gamble you'd be willing to take? Each year, Americans spend billions on diets that claim to promote weight loss, improve health, and quickly fix problems. The reality is that no high-quality studies lasting longer than five years indicate that most people can sustain significant weight loss, changes in body composition, and other major shifts through dieting. For the few individuals who do maintain weight loss, the cost is to become increasingly disordered and restrictive in their eating habits.

PSYCHOLOGICAL EFFECTS OF DIETING

* More self-criticism and greater shame
* Increased binging and more intense food cravings
* Higher risk of developing eating disorders or unhealthy eating habits
* A fixation on what you "can't" have, as well as anxiety around decisions related to food
* Social isolation or disengaging from social activities and interactions

PHYSICAL EFFECTS OF DIETING

* Weight gain—often more than you've lost (dieting is actually a consistent predictor of weight gain)
* Resistance to weight loss and conservation of body mass (your body thinks dieting is equivalent to famine)
* Higher risk of heart disease and premature death
* No longer being attuned to cues of hunger and fullness due to restrictive eating habits
* Irregular or skipped menstrual cycles
* Fertility issues (either now or in the future) caused by hormonal disruptions and regularly eating less than your body needs
* Higher risks of nutrition-related issues, including decreased bone mineral density; suboptimal intake of essential vitamins, minerals, or other nutrients; or increased sensitivity to high-fiber foods
* Impaired recovery after workouts, increased risk of injury, and/or delayed healing—especially when combined with compulsive exercise

THE ROLE OF REPETITION

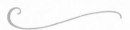

When you're dieting, there are long lists of foods you can't have. For whatever reason, they've been deemed "unhealthy" or "not allowed," but this creates more novelty and excitement around them. Your inner rebel, then, wants to push back against the rules and seek out these foods. This places certain foods on a pedestal, which can intensify cravings or set the stage for eating far past fullness when you finally allow yourself to have that particular food.

The common next step is to go back to avoiding that food, and the process repeats. With intuitive eating, the cycle breaks when you grant yourself permission to enjoy that food as much as you'd like (as uncomfortable as it may feel to do that). At first, you may feel afraid and out of control. But with support and persistence, repeated exposure makes the food less and less enticing. Eventually, you can become more habituated to ingredients and meals that were once forbidden.

Don't attempt this with all of your forbidden foods at once; that's a recipe for feeling overwhelmed, inadequate, or less confident with intuitive eating. Choose one item at a time, and reintroduce it in a manner that feels safe to you. If you're struggling, reach out to an intuitive eating professional, such as a dietitian or counselor, as you work through this process.

But if diets work as well as they claim to, why is there a constant stream of new ones? (Hint: They're often recycled or repackaged versions of diets that have fallen out of vogue.) Now more than ever, you have to be attuned to the sneaky ways dieting infiltrates the way you eat, shop, dress, cook, and live. As anti-diet dietitian Christy Harrison—an outspoken advocate for intuitive eating and host of the popular podcast, "Food Psych"—so aptly labeled it, diet culture is the "life thief" that robs you of your ability to fully participate in and enjoy life without the dark cloud of restriction or obsession.

Research supports a non-diet approach. If you really want to get serious about improving your health, it's time to shift your focus away from dieting's culture of No and ask what could happen if you embraced the world of Yes.

MY DIETING HISTORY

If you've attempted diets in the past, chances are you've learned a thing or two about them. It can be helpful to reflect on your history with dieting and, putting pounds lost aside, determine if they were actually successful.

Fill out the table that follows to the best of your memory. If needed, use your journal for additional space. It's okay to mourn the loss of dieting; it's often a familiar and predictable habit. But this exercise may help you realize that dieting has never delivered the results you've really wanted. Include any changes to your eating habits that excluded ingredients or an entire food group.

AGE OR YEAR _____	DIET OR HABIT_____		
Why did I start? Why did I stop?	Did it work? If so, were the results long-term?	Was there an element of exercise? If so, did I enjoy it?	What were the biggest downsides of this diet?

Other

AGE OR YEAR _____   DIET OR HABIT_____

Why did I start? Why did I stop?	Did it work? If so, were the results long-term?	Was there an element of exercise? If so, did I enjoy it?	What were the biggest downsides of this diet?

Other

AGE OR YEAR _____   DIET OR HABIT_____

Why did I start? Why did I stop?	Did it work? If so, were the results long-term?	Was there an element of exercise? If so, did I enjoy it?	What were the biggest downsides of this diet?

Other

AGE OR YEAR _____   DIET OR HABIT_____

Why did I start? Why did I stop?	Did it work? If so, were the results long-term?	Was there an element of exercise? If so, did I enjoy it?	What were the biggest downsides of this diet?

Other

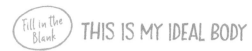

THIS IS MY IDEAL BODY

In the space that follows, draw a picture of your ideal body in terms of what it can do, how it provides for you, how it moves, and what it can do for others. Try to avoid including characteristics of physical appearance alone, and see how many ways you can dream of an ideal body that serves a purpose beyond looks alone. Likewise, ignore what you think an ideal body *should* look like or do; remember that all bodies are good bodies regardless of shape, size, ability, age, gender, or ethnicity.

Not feeling artistic? Not a problem. Use the space to write a few paragraphs (or more!) about what you envision.

The Hidden Costs of Restriction

People don't fail diets; diets fail people. Add that to their long list of draw-backs and hidden costs. These next exercises are intended to help you home in on the ways dieting has impacted your life.

 WHAT HAS DIETING TAKEN AWAY FROM YOU?

1. Dieting and building a lifestyle around restrictive food habits holds you back from life's richest experiences. What were some moments when dieting robbed you of your ability to enjoy or participate in an event? *Example: When I was on my most recent diet, I prepared different meals for my family while I ate only the food on my meal plan.*

    _____

    _____

2. How would those moments have looked had I given myself permission to participate? *Example: I could have enjoyed a meal with my family without leaving the table unsatisfied.*

    _____

    _____

3. How can I allow myself to participate in moments that I had abstained from in the past? *Example: I will prepare only one version of a meal for my entire family to enjoy and focus on the time we spend together instead of the nutrition in the meal.*

    _____

    _____

4. Now, put one of those suggestions you made for yourself previously into play. Don't be surprised if this experiment feels incredibly challenging and uncomfortable at first. Remember that it's common for your every thought to be preoccupied by food, especially if you're early in your journey toward intuitive eating. Keep your journal handy to record how your experiments go. As you begin the process of learning a new approach to eating, it's normal and acceptable to make mistakes or feel awkward.

OPERATING IN THE GRAY OF LIFE

Dieting is black and white in nature. Either you're "on a diet/off a diet" or "good/bad" or "doing it right/doing it wrong." It's human nature to create dichotomies like these. However, life is full of nuances that operate some-where in between this or that. Even in your own brain, it's natural to be feeling or thinking multiple things at once. Let's break open some of the nuances of a non-diet approach and step into the gray area by listing a few of your current thoughts. Whatever comes to mind is great, but start with "I feel . . . " or "I am . . . ". For example:

- I feel both the desire to be healthy—and to have peace of mind and happi-ness in my life.
- I want both to be confident in making food choices—and to have less guilt and judgment about what I eat.
- I am both strong and powerful—and I know my body sometimes needs time to relax/heal/recover.
- I know I can live as my authentic self—and I still struggle with accepting my body.

- _____

- _____

- _____

- _____

Review your list, and notice whether any judgments from your inner critic come up. Attempt to acknowledge them (I see you!) without reacting to them (But I'm not going to get into a debate with you!). Challenge yourself to notice these thoughts, and instead of responding harshly, adjust your tone as if you're speaking to yourself with the same compassion you might offer your best friend or a loved family member. Doing so is a kind way to quiet your inner critic as you reflect on what you've written. Add to your list as you notice more nuance within the context of your life.

Stop Fighting with Your Body

What if you responded to hunger like any other signal from your body? Imagine being able to address a physiological need using whatever's around. For instance, if you were in a car for a road trip and suddenly realized you needed to stop for gas, you'd most likely look for the nearest exit, take care of business, and start driving again. You'd do what you needed to do even if you had just stopped for the same reason earlier. Perhaps you'd be a little annoyed if now you're going to be late, but you wouldn't search for a reason to forgo stopping for gas. ("I don't think the gas gauge is really working. Maybe I need to distract myself or start pleading with the car to keep going.")

Likewise, if you were rushing to a meeting and had to use the stairs, you might get to the top and realize you feel winded. Instead of fighting your body, you'd likely take a few moments to catch your breath, compose yourself, and walk into the meeting when you were ready.

Although you may be highly aware of sensations like being out of breath, it's easy to lose connection to signals of hunger. You've been taught to ignore, numb, or distract yourself from the physical cues to eat. To reconnect with them, you have to recognize them again and relearn your best ways to respond. Often, it's as simple as eating something that is satisfying and filling.

TUNE INTO YOU

Those who score high on intuitive eating assessments also tend to score high in assessments for interoceptive awareness—the state of being mindfully aware. This shouldn't be surprising since intuitive eating helps you reconnect to your internal wisdom and base your decisions on internal cues and feedback versus external direction. That might mean:

* Noticing your heart starting to beat faster in response to something that makes you feel excited or anxious
* Feeling the sensation of the ground under your feet as you walk

- Knowing whether you feel hot or cold, and adjusting your environment or layers of clothing accordingly

Imagine how helpful this can be when applied to hunger and fullness. If you knew—and really trusted—the biological cues and physical sensations in your body, eating healthfully would be simpler. These next exercises are designed to help you tune into you.

 ## BODY SCAN MEDITATION

The body can carry tension and emotions in ways that aren't always apparent. Doing an easy body scan meditation can help identify where to invite more relaxation or gratitude into your body. Try this when you don't feel rushed (although you can also use it anytime you're stressed, anxious, or tense).

1. Start in a comfortable, quiet place, such as in a chair with your back supported and feet flat on the floor. Close your eyes.

2. Ground yourself by becoming aware of your breath, noticing how your chest rises and falls with each inhale and exhale.

3. Turn your focus to your toes. You don't have to do anything but notice where you feel tense or uncomfortable (if at all) in your toes as you inhale. As you exhale, picture the tension releasing or flowing out of that area.

4. Repeat the process, incrementally moving your focus up your lower legs, then your upper legs, hips, torso, chest, back, hands, arms, shoulders, neck, face, and the crown of your head.

5. When you're ready, slowly bring your awareness back to the space around you, and gently open your eyes.

If you find it challenging to concentrate on each area of the body in your mind's eye, try another form of a body scan meditation that incorporates physical touch.

1. Find a comfortable seated position in a quiet space, and close your eyes.

2. Place your right or left hand over your opposite wrist. Feel the weight of your hand against your skin.

3. Begin to slowly squeeze your wrist, increasing the pressure and noticing the sensations you feel. Hold your wrist tightly for 5 to 10 seconds, then gradually begin to release pressure, noticing how the sensation changes as you loosen your grip.

4. Repeat the process, working your way up your arm toward your shoulder. Take your time, and see how it feels as you focus your attention on each small part of the body.

5. Once you've reached your shoulder, switch sides and repeat this meditation on the opposite arm.

6. If there's any other area—such as the legs, feet, or neck—that's calling for some attention, go ahead and repeat the process there.

7. When you're ready, slowly bring your awareness back to the space around you, and gently open your eyes.

Afterward, notice whether you feel anything different in your body. Are some areas more relaxed than when you started? Has your stress level decreased? Are there any other sensations? In the space that follows, circle or write down anything noteworthy. Practice this meditation as a simple way to ground yourself if you ever feel the need to check in with your body at any time.

BODY PART	EMOTION	PHYSICAL OBSERVATIONS
Neck	Tension	Sharp pain
Shoulders	Stress	Tingling
Throat	Anxiety	Sore
Back	Discomfort	Throbbing
Stomach	Fear	Queasy
Chest	Gratitude or connection	Relaxed
Hands	Anger or disappointment	Weakness
Head	Happiness or contentment	Lightness

QUIT THE BODY-CHECKING GAME

Another way to tune into your body is to reduce how often you compare it to either your past body, your ideal body, or other people's bodies. The game of comparison is a slippery slope toward dissatisfaction and a return to dieting. Body checking can look like:

- Scanning the room when you first walk in to see who has the largest/smallest/fittest/most attractive frame
- Glancing in the mirror every chance you get
- Adjusting clothing to create the illusion of thinness
- Repeatedly looking at your body to check that you don't appear bloated, soft, and so on
- Repeatedly touching parts of your body about which you feel uncomfortable
- Stepping on the scale one or more times a day

This exercise is meant to challenge the way you view human bodies and perhaps confront a bias for thinness. Play an episode of your favorite TV show or a clip from a movie. Find a scene with multiple characters and hit pause.

- What are my first impressions of their appearances?

_____

- Am I making assumptions about the characters based on their appearances?

_____

- Which stereotypes are being portrayed here? Are they accurate? Do I agree or disagree with them?

_____

- Does this scene represent how the real world looks? Do the actors showcase a wide range of body sizes and types?

_____

- Next, describe your body objectively and neutrally, without attaching either positive or negative meaning to it.

I notice . . .

_____

I think . . .

_____

I feel . . .

_____

I sense . . .

_____

My body can . . .

_____

My body is . . .

_____

Tip: The next time you catch yourself engaging in body-checking behavior, pause and make a statement of gratitude or acknowledgment to your body. It doesn't have to be overly gleeful, but attempt to tell yourself something that's not rooted in hate or disrespect toward your body. Here are some examples:

- You catch your reflection in a mirror and are uncomfortable with what you see. You can say, "I notice that my body looks different than I expected it to today."
- You're very aware of the folds of your belly as you sit in your jeans. You can say, "My belly is part of my body, and my body is my home. It holds my organs and my spirit. It is allowed to exist and gives me a place in this world."
- You've changed outfits six times this morning because you dislike how things are fitting. You can say, "My body deserves to wear clothes that fit well and are comfortable to move in. The size on the tag doesn't define my worth, so if I need to change sizes, I will. My body deserves to be comfortable."

Trade Punishment for Compassion

At this point, things should look more gray than black and white. You've begun to trade punishment and compensation for more curiosity and compassion around how you eat and look at your body. You're exchanging the rules someone else wrote for you for something rooted in your strengths and values.

This stuff isn't easy, but there's no shame in recognizing any struggles that have come up along the way. If you're aiming for truly sustainable changes, it may help to focus on your strengths and rally around the things that seem more natural or intuitive. After all, there's plenty of time to work on the tougher areas while you continue to rebuild body trust and confidence. These next exercises can help you strengthen your self-compassion and remove judgments.

JOURNAL: *It's common to say unkind things to yourself that you wouldn't dare say aloud to someone else. One small step toward self-compassion is speaking to yourself as you would a child. By seeing yourself as a kid, you can start rewriting the narrative you believe. Spend some time writing a letter to yourself at age six. What would you tell that version of you? How would you encourage and empower them for the future? If you have time, try writing a letter to yourself at age 90. Observe how your inner critic recedes and gets quieter as you focus on what you really value.*

Practice

EXTENDING COMPASSION TO OTHERS

In some ways, cultivating self-compassion requires training just like a new skill or sport. It can feel awkward or difficult to be so kind to yourself, especially if you've become numb to your needs or body. Because self-compassion is intimately tied to compassion for others, this exercise is designed to help you strengthen your capacity in creative ways.

Use this BINGO card to increase your ability to be kind to others. There's no time limit; fill it in as opportunities arise. In the blank squares, write something you think would invite more kindness into your routine.

Offer a compliment to someone whose body is similar to yours. Instead of focusing on appearance, compliment an action you saw them do or their character.	_____ _____ _____ _____	Gift an enjoyable experience to someone. It doesn't need to be expensive or extravagant, but ideally it should be something they otherwise would not gift themselves.
_____ _____ _____ _____	Run an errand or help someone who's overwhelmed or struggling. Sometimes a small act is all they need.	Schedule time to connect with a close friend or family member. Make it known that you value the relationship and appreciate the effort they make to stay connected.
Celebrate someone else's accomplishment (major or minor, professional or personal), and tell them how proud you are of what they've achieved.	Make eye contact or acknowledge someone's presence as you greet or thank them, even if they're a stranger.	_____ _____ _____ _____

After a few BINGOs, consider what it would be like to be on the receiving end of those kind acts. Do you believe you deserve to be treated with the same compassion? Are you waiting for others to extend this to you? Are you comfortable creating that culture of compassion in your life? If not, what are some of the roadblocks that make it feel challenging?

_____

_____

_____

_____

Remember that all bodies are good bodies; your appearance does not negate the fact that you, too, are deserving of kindness. If you aren't in a place where you can extend it to yourself, scan your community for support—perhaps a coworker, sibling, partner, or friend. Even having a conversation about what you need to feel supported is a sweet way to remind yourself that you're not alone on your intuitive eating journey.

Takeaways

- Dieting harms your psychological and physical health in many ways. Reflecting on your history with food may reveal how diets and other food habits have failed you.

- You have a chance to get reacquainted with your body by checking in with its physical and emotional sensations. A simple body scan meditation or listening closely to subtle body cues can rebuild trust and connection.

- You're not likely to respect or care for something you hate. Offering compassion and kindness to yourself is a difficult but important part of healing your relationship with food and your body.

CHAPTER THREE

Listen to Your BODY

DIETS OFFER A CONVENIENT (although not ideal) way to outsource some of the decision-making around food. They give you a reprieve from the sometimes exhausting tasks of planning meals, choosing ingredients, or knowing when and how much to eat. It's easy to see how you can convince yourself that food rules really are sustainable and that the lifestyles they prescribe can be easily maintained. In reality, dieting guidelines dampen your awareness of the body's nourishment need signals.

What's Your Body Trying to Tell You?

Hunger isn't something to be feared or mistrusted, but if you were once convinced that eating should be restrained, careful, limited, or controlled, you may question whether you are physically hungry and give less thought to feeling truly full and satisfied.

Dieting also plants a seed of entitlement and obligation around eating. And why wouldn't it? If there are meal plans or food rules telling you how much to eat, it's implied that anything more than that must be overeating (even if it's less than what your body needs). Here are a few examples of how some programs cleverly instruct how to eat instead of letting you determine it for yourself:

- Joining or staying in the "clean plate club" and always finishing every last bite of a meal—even if you don't like the food or already feel full—simply because it's written into the diet plan
- Choosing diet versions of foods—things like natural, fat-free, or no-sugar-added desserts—frequently or in large amounts because they're perceived as being "healthier"

- Eating low-cal "air food" in order to trick yourself into fullness. (Think: rice cakes, plain popcorn, non-starchy vegetables, diet soda, black coffee, lemon water, or other zero-calorie beverages)*
- Snacking throughout the day on portion-controlled packs or "allowed" foods**

Think back to the earlier example on page 29 of running up a flight of stairs; it seems almost ridiculous to question something as natural as hunger. Yet, that's exactly what so many people do, often to the point that they're eating in a mindless state of autopilot much of the time and lamenting the times when they finally notice their hunger again. As uncomfortable and challenging as it may be, getting familiar with your body can help you understand what it's really trying to tell you.

NO ONE KNOWS YOUR BODY AS WELL AS YOU DO

Intuitive eating strives to reestablish you as the expert of your body. You're the only one who calls it home, so you're the authority on what's going on inside. Even a health care professional with lots of experience doesn't have as much experience with your body as you do. They can share objective information, evidence-based recommendations, and clinical knowledge, but they aren't aware of the intimate details of your lifestyle, all of your likes and dislikes, and how you experience the world.

You're also the only one who can advocate for your body to get what it needs. Part of becoming a more informed and empowered eater is speaking up by saying, "Actually, I need something else," or "I really don't want this." You and you alone have the ability to say exactly what you need or want from eating, and getting in touch with your hunger and satiety cues may be one place to start.

---

* If you eat "air foods" because you truly like them, by all means, enjoy. Just be aware of whether you're relying only on these foods. Would you eat them even if you weren't aware of how few calories they had?

**If portion-controlled, single-serving packs make life easier (for example, when you are traveling or running errands), they're a great option. Just be aware of whether you're limiting yourself or experiencing restrictive thoughts that make you feel like you're only allowed to eat a single, predetermined portion.

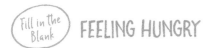

FEELING HUNGRY

Sensations of hunger and fullness are not black and white—there is a whole range, from overly hungry to overly full. Either end of that spectrum can be equally uncomfortable, but the middle is, well, just right.

OVERLY HUNGRY	Intense, urgent, and painful hunger
	Ravenous, irritable, and anxious to eat
	Very hungry and looking forward to eating
NORMAL EATING RANGE	Ready to eat; hunger is manageable but not urgent
	Slightly hungry
	Neutral; not hungry or full
	Starting to feel the signs of fullness
	Comfortably full; feeling satisfied and content
OVERLY FULL	Unpleasantly full but not uncomfortable physically
	Too full and uncomfortable
	Painfully full or stuffed; possibly nauseous

That said, it's all subjective; what feels like extreme hunger or fullness to you might be moderate to your best friend. Even the same meal or serving size can affect fullness differently from one meal to the next, so don't be surprised if the lunch you always pack gets you to a comfortable level of fullness one day but leaves you hungry and searching for more another. Use the hunger spectrum and table that follows to check your hunger throughout a day (make a copy or recreate it in your journal if it's something you want to do again and again). Track every couple of hours while you're awake or simply when you remember, writing about the level of hunger you're experiencing, along with anything else you notice.

TIME	HUNGER LEVEL	WHAT DO I FEEL IN MY BODY?

FEELING FULL

Tracking your fullness is just as important as your hunger. Fill out the table that follows before, during, and after a meal or snack. Don't worry about completing everything (that's neither realistic nor necessary), but if you happen to be thinking about it, you may see some interesting patterns for how your hunger shifts to fullness throughout a meal. Practice this for various meals at different times and in different settings. You don't have to write down every detail; making mental notes or simply checking in with yourself can be just as insightful.

TIME	HOW HUNGRY AM I?	WHAT DO I FEEL IN MY BODY?	HOW SATISFIED AM I?
1 hour before eating, grocery shopping, or ordering food			
While food is cooking			
When you start eating			
5 minutes later			
15 minutes later			
1 hour later			

There may be times you can't accurately determine these things. That's okay. Remember to let go of judgments as much as possible and take on the role of a neutral observer who's simply curious to learn more. The point is to simply look for patterns: Are you often overly full an hour after eating? If so, you might want to make adjustments to your meals. Are you often still hungry an hour after the dishes are done? Consider adding something to your meals to help you feel more satisfied.

AM I A DISTRACTED EATER?

Defaulting to mindlessness is a common state in this hectic world. Are you accustomed to simply going through the motions? Or have you fallen into a routine that doesn't allow you to be actively aware of your actions? While mindfulness applies to all aspects of life, for the purposes of this workbook, you'll focus on how to cultivate a more mindful eating experience.

Distractions are not necessarily problematic; in fact, it's extremely rare to have a meal that is devoid of external stimuli. Besides, wouldn't it feel a little bit awkward without something happening in the background? It's normal to feel uncomfortable when left alone with your own thoughts. At the family dinner table, a busy restaurant, or a loud public place, the opportunities to have a completely tranquil, mindful eating experience are few and far between.

However, frequent or repeated distractions can cause you to neglect your hunger and satiety cues and contribute to mindless eating. For this exercise, consider the items in the following table and think about how often they appear in your eating routine. Then, see if you notice any patterns about which distractions come up most often.

DISTRACTION	TIME OF DAY AND MEAL	DISTRACTION LEVEL*	AM I EATING ALONE OR WITH PEOPLE?
Reading a book, newspaper, or magazine			
Checking social media			
Reading on a desktop, tablet, or smartphone			
Playing a game on my phone or tablet			
Watching a TV show or movie on television			
Watching a TV show or movie on my phone or tablet			
Eating in my car			
Eating in the living room			
Eating in my office or at my desk			
Eating while walking or physically moving			
Eating during a presentation, training, or other event			
Eating during a conversation with one or more other people			
Eating while doing chores or housework			

*(on a scale of 0 to 10; 0 is fully present and 10 is completely distracted)

DISTRACTION	TIME OF DAY AND MEAL	DISTRACTION LEVEL*	AM I EATING ALONE OR WITH PEOPLE?
Eating on the job or while trying to complete a task			
Texting or messaging other people			
Talking on the phone			
Driving			
Checking my email or messages			
Making or reviewing my to-do list			
Caring for children or other family members			

From here, you can decide which of these distractions to tackle. As you've learned, distractions are not necessarily a problem. In fact, if you can accurately tune in to your hunger and fullness signals in the presence of diversions like the ones listed above, you might not need to make any changes. But if they interfere with your awareness of hunger and fullness, you might want to devote some time to creating a more sacred space around eating.

Eating Mindfully

Intuitive eating is often oversimplified as "eat when you're hungry; stop when you're full." Mindful eating can also be overly generalized. What does "mindful eating" mean to you? Do you immediately think of engaging with all five senses as you're chewing? That's part of it, of course, but there are many more aspects. Sure, it can be helpful to bring awareness to how foods taste, feel, smell, sound, and look. But its other benefits include:

- Identifying your true food preferences when it comes to flavors, textures, serving styles, or temperatures
- Recognizing there's no right or wrong way to eat, and removing judgment from your food choices
- Accepting your unique food choices
- Being more conscious or present during meals
- Becoming aware of how your food choices align with your unique values or support your version of health and well-being
- Understanding how food choices impact other people, your community, and the larger food system

While there can be many interpretations of mindfulness as it relates to eating, here are some ways you can apply it:

- Choosing foods that are satisfying, both physically and emotionally or psychologically, for all five senses. After all, it's a challenge to be mindful if it involves food you dislike or don't find satisfying.
- Considering the positive and nourishing aspects of all food, based on taste and your health or how they make you feel.
- Allowing yourself to have food preferences, and not judging your choices. You enjoy some foods more than others, right? There are also probably some you dislike or feel neutral or indifferent toward. They may change over time or look different than someone else's preferences. Removing this judgment—especially about things that have been given a health halo—is an often overlooked area of mindful eating.
- Acknowledging your hunger and fullness cues. Again, notice them, but resist the urge to judge them.
- Allowing those cues to guide your decisions about when and how much you eat, instead of relying on external cues like a meal plan, time of day, or calories.

BRINGING AWARENESS TO YOUR LIKES AND DISLIKES

Tuning into your senses can offer clues about what you truly enjoy (or don't enjoy) about eating. When you're dieting, you may often overlook your preferences or set them aside for the sake of following a meal plan or prescriptive approach. This leads to disappointing meals, where you may feel full but still feel distracted by thoughts of food or eating. The next time you pause to eat, ask yourself:

* Do I like the flavor of this food? Does it need more or less saltiness, acidity, sweetness, spiciness, etc.? Can I adjust this food to make it more enjoyable?
* Do I like the texture? Do I wish it were more/less crunchy? Chewy? Sticky? How many other ways could I describe the texture?
* Do I like the temperature? Would I like this more/less if it were another time of year (for example, eating hot soup in winter rather than summer)? What about my drink? Would I prefer it to be hot or cold?
* Do I like how this food looks? Is it important for my food to be colorful and vibrant? Does it need to be nicely arranged? Or does that not matter to me?
* Do I like how filling this is? Do I need something hearty to fill me up, or would I prefer something lighter?

As you can see, tuning into your senses goes far beyond simple taste or smell.

BRINGING AWARENESS TO YOUR SATISFACTION

Your responses to the questions in the previous section can help you become more aware of what satisfies you. Simply eating enough or the correct types of food should get the job done, right? In reality, you may not have had what you were really craving. When dieting, it's common to sacrifice satisfaction or engage in some kind of performative eating. You might compare it to eating out of obligation, either to your diet, to someone who prepared the food, or to the people who may be watching you eat. You may have felt obligated to uphold the unrealistic or unsustainable expectations you placed on yourself. In reality, none of those obligatory eating practices makes for a mindful eating experience. So ask yourself this question: Is it worth it to continue being unsatisfied?

HABIT BUILDER

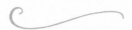

Listening to your body is easier said than done in a world that encourages dissatisfaction and disconnection. Part of building resilience to this involves the curious questioning of what you believe or think when you notice you're comparing your body to others or what you think you "should" be doing. Start small by challenging these thoughts and beliefs as they arise. Here are some things to ask yourself:

- How does my body feel right now? What could I do to support the way I want to feel in my body?
- Would I still do this activity if no one was watching? Am I doing it because I hope that my body will change?
- What is my body really trying to tell me? Am I prepared to listen to it, or do I still feel compelled to eat or move a certain way?

Focus on the behaviors you habituated while you were dieting. From there, consider questioning or challenging the beliefs and thoughts underlying those behaviors—or think about what an alternative behavior might look like. Eventually, you can explore some of those alternatives and see how you feel using the mindfulness techniques from this chapter. Some may even turn into positive habits.

BRINGING AWARENESS TO YOUR EATING ENVIRONMENT

You can apply mindfulness to more than just your food. How often have you paused to consider the setting of your meals or snacks? It can be interesting to notice how your perception of satisfaction and fullness changes depending on the setting. For example, a woman says she doesn't like fast food, but she eats it anyway. She says the food is hot, savory, and tastes good, but it isn't filling. She often feels hungry again a short time later, plus she doesn't like how it affects her energy levels. Yet she still eats it on a regular basis and even looks forward to those meals. After digging a little deeper, she connects the dots to realize that these are some of the only meals she eats alone, away from her desk and the stress of her job and responsibilities at home. Although the food itself isn't very fulfilling, she savors being able to eat in a completely different environment, by herself.

If you notice there is tension, stress, or chaos surrounding your meals, mindfulness may help you reconsider your eating environment. It's not always possible to completely change; that's not the point of mindfulness. But mindfulness can help reduce judgment toward your food choices or eating environment and shift your focus to something else instead.

BRINGING AWARENESS TO REPLACEMENT FOODS

Think about some of the food choices you've made while dieting. Have you ever selected foods based on their perceived health benefits or how they're marketed? Have you opted for a food that is a so-called safe or healthier version of what you really want? You're not alone. These placeholder foods are a swap for the foods you actually crave. Think about granola or protein bars. Say there's one marketed as a healthy choice that aligns with your diet, so you bought it. It's somewhat sweet, a little bit chewy, and pretty tasty (so you think)—it's even named after a familiar sweet treat like chocolate chip cookie dough or peanut butter cups. Because you allow yourself to have this type of bar, you catch yourself binge-eating the entire box—it's one of the few sweet things you can have. But, as you start to implement intuitive eating habits and learn about what you do and don't like, you may realize that you don't actually enjoy these bars. When you give yourself permission to have other sweet things, like a peanut butter cup instead of the protein bar stand-in, the bar's flavor and texture may no longer appeal to you. That's because they were simply a placeholder for what you really wanted to eat but didn't allow yourself to have.

This is just one example of how being more mindful about eating can help you learn which foods you truly enjoy and which foods you eat because you think they're healthy. In fact, with a little mindfulness, certain replacement foods suddenly lose their appeal. The following exercises aim to bring more mindfulness and awareness to how and what you eat.

HOW AM I DOING?

Perhaps you're already using mindfulness to focus during meals or explore other aspects of eating. But mindfulness and gentle, nonjudgmental awareness can benefit you beyond the kitchen table.

Periodically checking in with yourself to ask, "How am I doing?" is similar to the body scan meditation you practiced earlier on page 30. In this case, instead of noticing physical sensations, take note of thoughts or emotions at any given moment. You don't have to label or categorize them, though you might recognize them as positive, negative, or indifferent. Nothing needs to be done with those emotions. You're simply saying, "Yep, I see sadness there. Oh, and now here comes a little anxiety." At the very least, it's worth celebrating anytime you notice them—or even feel compelled to act on them—but didn't allow them to interfere with your ability to take care of yourself. Each time this happens, you continue to build resilience and be less triggered by negative thoughts or emotions the next time they inevitably pop up.

During your next meal, record in your journal anything noteworthy or relevant that comes to mind as you eat—even for just a minute. Gradually work your way up to longer stretches of time, or repeat this process more often throughout the day until it becomes easier and more intuitive to pause and check with yourself.

Build Body Awareness

Bringing mindfulness into your daily routine applies to more than just eating. Dieting often teaches you to numb or ignore the signals you feel within your body. That's why you may ignore a grumbling stomach, a sore body part during a workout, or the exhausted brain that begs for a break. There may be moments in your day when you forget about your body entirely and something (like pain or a loud noise) suddenly snaps your awareness back to the fact that you do, indeed, need to take care of yourself. How often do you realize:

- You're clenching your jaw or grinding your teeth?
- Your shoulders are tensed up near your ears?
- You feel GI symptoms due to anxiety or something you ate?
- You stayed up later than usual and suddenly feel exhausted?
- You have been ignoring an ache or pain, only to bump against something or otherwise be reminded of it?
- You've become accustomed to constant headaches, backaches, or joint pain?
- You've been wearing clothes that bind or constrict and don't allow you to move as freely as you want?
- You've been in the same position for so long, a hand or foot has fallen asleep?

It might seem like this stuff would be common sense, but it's easy to become a pro at ignoring the obvious until you consciously pay attention to it. The following exercises are intended to help you build or rebuild body awareness.

MINDFUL MOVEMENT

Bodies are meant to move. In fact, most people are constantly moving all day long, from getting up and brushing teeth to walking into work and washing the dishes. These routine tasks are opportunities to bring attention to the way you feel. How does your body physically feel during the following activities? Once these actions are accomplished, do you feel the way you'd like to in your body? If there are other activities that you regularly engage in, feel free to add those to this list.

- Getting out of bed _____
- Sitting in a chair at a table _____
- Sitting on a sofa, couch, or recliner _____
- Getting in and out of a car or vehicle _____
- Walking up a flight of stairs _____
- Standing in the shower or sitting in the bathtub _____
- Taking a deep breath and exhaling slowly _____
- _____
- _____
- _____
- _____
- _____
- _____
- _____

Ready to Start Moving?

As you transition to a more mindful, intuitive approach to eating, a temporary break from exercise or structured movement might be appropriate. Food and movement are intricately connected, and you may notice you have a history of starting a new exercise routine every time you've started a new diet.

Movement is often overcomplicated, but it doesn't have to be. Your body was meant to move—whether that be walking, running, climbing, or moving around things in your environment. When you don't, not only is it harder to maintain everyday activity, but you can become that much more out of touch with your physical self.

In today's modern world (and after you outgrow organized sports or playgrounds), physical movement and enjoyable activities often get phased out in favor of structured or sometimes monotonous exercise routines that don't always elicit the same playful energy you had on the monkey bars or soccer field. That means you may give more credence to what you think you "should" be doing instead of relying on internal cues.

Just like some foods, certain movements can be a good fit for some but not others. If you have to make sacrifices in order to fit in prescribed or rigid fitness plans, or it begins to disrupt your life or add stress and anxiety, you may need to back off from exercise for a time. Consulting with an intuitive eating dietitian or therapist can guide you when deciding to start working out again or when there is still work to be done to heal your relationship with exercising.

JOURNAL: What would you like to change about how you feel during these activities? How could healthy behaviors help you with that? Example: Finding a form of gentle movement might help my joints ache less, and I could get in and out of the car more easily and with less pain.

But, this is only temporary; a regular fitness routine, even a very gentle one, can coexist alongside intuitive eating. In fact, it's part of the process.

MOVING MEDITATION

If you're craving a little movement or want to adopt a mindful, conscious approach to being more active, start with a simple moving meditation like this one. If you're not sure whether you've reached this point yet, working with a dietitian, therapist, or personal trainer with experience in intuitive eating can help you determine if the time is right.

A temporary break from planned activity is essential to reframing your views and beliefs about exercise, whether you're recovering from an injury, illness, or simply learning to be more comfortable in your body. If mobility is difficult for you, know that this exercise is optional. Honoring your health and respecting your body means understanding your limits and choosing to access physical activity in a way that's helpful. It should not leave you feeling so depleted that you have no energy left for other things, nor should it create stress, discomfort, or pain.

To be clear, a moving or walking meditation is not intended to improve fitness or leave you sweaty or winded. It's a simple way to invite more awareness and strengthen a mind-body connection.

1. Find an open, flat space where you can take 8 to 10 steps. If you'd like, and if the setting allows, you can even remove your shoes and socks to better connect to the ground.

2. As you begin to walk, notice your posture, pace, balance, and the sensation of your feet lifting and reconnecting to the ground as you move.

3. When you've gone 8 to 10 steps, turn around and retrace your steps. You might choose to focus on your breath, counting your steps, or a short mantra or thought.

4. Once you've completed your meditation, jot down any feelings that came up in your journal.

Takeaways

- No one knows your body as well as you do, but you may need to spend some time learning your body's signals and rebuilding awareness.

- Tracking your hunger and fullness can bring a lot of insight about how and why you eat, and what it takes for you to feel satisfied and full.

- Mindful eating is a part of intuitive eating, but it's much more than simply slowing down and chewing your food. Remember that you cannot mindfully eat your way to food freedom.

- Mindfulness is also helpful with movement and noticing how your body feels. Start getting curious about observing the way your body feels throughout the day, as well as during exercise.

CHAPTER FOUR

FEED Your HUNGER

PHYSICAL HUNGER IS BORN FROM A PHYSIOLOGICAL NEED. It's your body's way of saying, "Feed me!" or "I need some energy!" But it's rarely that simple. That's why it's important to also consider emotional hunger—times you feel driven to eat out of curiosity to taste a new food, find comfort, or mask uncomfortable emotions. Neither physical nor emotional hunger is "wrong" or "bad," and you can even experience both at the same time. You'll learn more about emotional eating in this chapter as you learn how to identify hunger versus feelings.

The connection between the body and mind is a powerful thing. Even if you haven't given much thought to it in the past, you've likely experienced butterflies in your stomach when you're apprehensive or nervous. You've also likely experienced sweaty palms or flushed cheeks during a heated argument. Being aware of these things is a part of emotional intelligence, meaning that you can identify or name what you're feeling. But despite the fact that you know you need something in those moments, how often do you express that? And how often do you act on it?

The Body-Mind Connection

Suppressing thoughts or needs is known as self-silencing. It can have a negative impact on mental health and result in depressive symptoms or disordered eating behaviors. Research suggests that many women first experience self-silencing during adolescence. If you think back to your younger years, what is your first memory of not asking for something you needed or wanted? These unvoiced needs may be held in your mind and become internalized whether they're true or not. And since food offers a way to self-soothe or try to regulate these needs, your relationship with food can become even more distraught as a result. Throw a diet on top of all that, and oh boy.

On the flip side, combining aspects of emotional awareness, intuitive eating, and voicing your needs can yield significant benefits for your health. Expression of needs is also a way to start living out the values you identified in chapter 1 (page 10). When you recognize what's happening in your body or how you're feeling—and are then able to voice it or act on it—you're reinforcing that you can take good care of yourself. You no longer have to rely on external food rules or dieting; you are confident that regardless of what situation you find yourself in, you're able to provide what you need.

Although this is a relatively simple solution, it is far from easy. This is where many people struggle with getting on board with intuitive eating. You can intellectually understand that intuitive eating and the rejection of dieting are helpful. But it can be difficult to navigate the nuanced ways it applies to life.

If you find yourself facing those same questions, you aren't alone. The journey to becoming an intuitive eater is rarely (if ever) linear. You may circle around the idea for weeks, months, or even years before you feel fully prepared to implement it into your life. If this sounds like you, working through some of your thoughts, feelings, and beliefs about it may bring clarity and the courage to move forward.

You Can't "Fix" Your Feelings

Dieting can be comfortable because of the way it builds community and connection. There are meetings, online forums, and prompts to share results on social media. Even if it's superficial—say, friends you met at the gym because you all started a similar diet around the same time—it's nice to feel accepted and supported. It's okay to acknowledge that that feels good. Although you've learned that dieting is not helpful for good health in the long run, it's serving a purpose for you at that point in time.

It's hard to leave those communities, especially, if they involve challenging the authority of a health care professional or explaining it time and again to friends or family. Stepping into that discomfort can be, well, incredibly uncomfortable. And it's bound to stir up even more feelings in addition to whatever you're already noticing about food or your body. All are valid, and they're all connected to something. That may be an event from your past or something that's happening now. It could be uncertainty about the future or your fears and anxieties. None of your feelings are wrong or need to change. It can be enough to recognize them and name them as being highly uncomfortable.

But a strong aversion to dealing with feelings (and, thus, avoiding them) can impair your ability to take care of yourself. Sometimes it manifests as emotional eating, which can often feel scary to acknowledge or talk about. Emotional eating can also serve as the scapegoat for feeling out of control around food. You may have even labeled yourself an emotional eater, and confronting something you've incorporated into your identity can be incredibly difficult.

EMOTIONAL EATING ISN'T ALWAYS A BAD THING

Experts and the media often tout emotional eating as a bad thing that needs to be managed. However, intuitive eating appreciates the comforting and emotional aspects of food and invites you to openly grant permission to enjoy the experience of eating. In fact, there are just as many positive or neutral reasons to eat as there are negative. Denying the emotional response to eat a favorite meal is really just another form of the self-silencing mentioned at the beginning of this chapter (see page 58).

So the question isn't necessarily "How can I stop emotional eating?" but "Do I want to?" There's an entire spectrum of human emotion connected to what we put on our plates. Do you really want to write that off or disregard those feelings entirely? Or could you become more comfortable with those that seem anything less than positive?

Emotional eating is only a problem if it interferes with the choices you make and causes friction in your relationship with food. It's a coping mechanism that stems from diet culture. In previous generations, there was very little judgment or even awareness of using food in this way, and there are low levels of emotional eating in places absent of a diet culture.

You may be asking yourself: "Is this a problem for me, personally?" This question might have to do with the frequency or degree to which you use food to cope with your feelings. Your discomfort with emotional eating or identifying as an emotional eater can stem from the judgment that diet culture casts on those who can't maintain the high standards and expectations of dieting. If, however, no one was watching the way you use food to feel a certain way, would you still have a problem with it?

If your answer is no, perhaps there isn't much that needs to be done. But if you still feel like you'd rather address it and explore alternative ways to cope, a non-diet approach can help. These next exercises will move you closer to a place where you're no longer simply feeding your emotions.

EMOTIONAL EATING REFLECTION

Use the chart that follows to reflect on the last time you remember an emotional connection to something you ate. Consider both the positive and negative emotions that you associated with the experience. If the details escape you, you can simply check the box. Reflect on your responses, and consider ways that you can cultivate the feelings you want. It may offer valuable insight into whether there are settings or activities you've been avoiding or limiting, or perhaps where setting some boundaries may be appropriate.

MEMORY OR EXPERIENCE WITH FOOD	EMOTION	HOW OFTEN DOES THIS HAPPEN?
	Frustration or resentment	
	Stress or anxiety	
	Celebration or excitement	
	Anger	
	Sadness	
	Loneliness	
	Boredom	
	Nostalgia	
	Happiness	

Which emotions do I experience most often with food or while eating?

_____

Which emotions do I experience least often?

_____

Which (if any) emotions do I never experience?

_____

Which emotions would I like to experience?

_____

FIRST: WHAT AM I CRAVING?

It's normal to sometimes ignore the full range of emotions and simplify them to say you feel "sad," "angry," or "bored." But, oftentimes, these oversimplifications are masking something much deeper and more complex, and certain compulsions can shed light on what you need to do to let that emotion go. In some cases, it may be food. Other times, it's a craving for something that food can't offer. The worksheet that follows can be completed in less than 5 minutes; use it the next time you're craving something or feel compelled to eat for a reason not related to hunger.

Date and Time: _____

Is this true, physical hunger? _____

Refer back to the hunger gradient on page 41. Where is my physical hunger

right now? _____

Food craving: _____

What's so special about this food? _____

What's going on? What is the trigger? _____

_____

SECOND: HOW DO I FEEL?

afraid	distressed	irritated	self-conscious
agitated	disturbed	jealous	sensitive
agony	embarrassed	lonely	shaky
angry	exhausted	longing	shocked
annoyed	fatigued	lost	shy
anxious	fragile	marginalized	sick
ashamed	frustrated	miserable	sleepy
bored	furious	nervous	stressed
burned out	grief	overwhelmed	surprised
concerned	guilty	pain	suspicious
confused	hateful	panicked	tense
contempt	heartbroken	pity	torn
cranky	heavyhearted	puzzled	self-conscious
depressed	helpless	regretful	unhappy
devastated	hesitant	rejected	uninterested
disappointed	hopeless	remorseful	upset
disconnected	horrified	resentful	vulnerable
discouraged	hostile	reserved	weak
disgusted	hurt	restless	worried
displeased	impatient	sad	
distracted	insecure	scared	

THIRD: WHAT DO I REALLY NEED?

Physical well-being

- ☐ comfort, warmth
- ☐ fresh air
- ☐ movement/exercise
- ☐ safety
- ☐ sexual expression
- ☐ sleep
- ☐ sunshine/daylight
- ☐ touch
- ☐ water

Harmony

- ☐ beauty
- ☐ comfort, warmth
- ☐ fresh air
- ☐ justice/fairness
- ☐ movement/exercise
- ☐ order
- ☐ peace
- ☐ predictability
- ☐ relaxation
- ☐ safety
- ☐ sexual expression
- ☐ sleep
- ☐ stability

Connection

- ☐ acceptance
- ☐ appreciation
- ☐ belonging, community
- ☐ care, affection
- ☐ closeness, intimacy
- ☐ communication
- ☐ compassion
- ☐ consistency
- ☐ cooperation
- ☐ hearing (hear/be heard)
- ☐ information, knowledge
- ☐ love
- ☐ respect
- ☐ seeing (see/be seen)
- ☐ support

Meaning

- ☐ awareness
- ☐ challenge, to be challenged
- ☐ clarity
- ☐ contribution
- ☐ creativity
- ☐ empowerment
- ☐ hope
- ☐ inspiration
- ☐ purpose
- ☐ self-confidence
- ☐ to matter

Autonomy

- ☐ choice
- ☐ freedom
- ☐ independence

Honesty

- ☐ authenticity
- ☐ integrity
- ☐ transparency

Play

- ☐ adventure
- ☐ celebration
- ☐ diversity, something different
- ☐ fun
- ☐ humor, laughter
- ☐ lightness
- ☐ passion
- ☐ relaxation
- ☐ spontaneity
- ☐ variety

Can food give me what I need?

_____

_____

_____

How would eating this food make my body feel?

_____

_____

_____

What can I do instead to satisfy my real need?

_____

_____

_____

Keep in mind that even if you complete this exercise, you're still allowed to eat the food you are craving. Mindful and intuitive eating doesn't mean you must deny yourself the food you desire; it simply means you have more opportunity to consider other factors before making your decision. Intuitive eating grants the unconditional permission to eat (and enjoy!) food, so even if you determine that there's an emotional reason for your craving and that the food you want will not address the emotion, you're still absolutely entitled to eat that food if you want to.

Getting Friendly with Your Feelings

What would happen if you invited more emotions into your life? Could you become more comfortable with the ones you're averse to and more appreciative of the ones you're attracted to? Casting certain emotions in a negative or destructive light is like labeling foods as "bad" or "unhealthy." In some cases, those things are appropriate, necessary, or perhaps the only options. Labeling and dismissing emotions isn't a helpful strategy because no single emotion can replace another. They have purposes to serve, such as:

- Feeling fear alerts you to a threat, just like feeling happiness makes you smile.
- Feeling anxiety will tell you that you need to prepare.
- Feeling sadness won't lead to contentment or ease, but it might indicate something in your life isn't working out.

With intuitive eating, food has less power to control you, and you are more equipped to look at it objectively as a tool that supports you. Likewise, you can start seeing your emotions as messengers or information updates. Emotions are important because they keep you aware of what's going on, and that's critical for your safety and well-being. Although we aren't facing the same threats we encountered thousands of years ago, our emotions continue to keep us healthy and happy in our modern world.

The following exercises show how your emotions are informative and when you can start calling out self-limiting or judgmental thoughts.

HABIT BUILDER

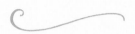

Getting carried away with emotions, especially in the heat of the moment, is a part of life. It's sometimes easy to blow things out of proportion or give too much credence to your emotions without reflecting on whether they're rooted in reality.

Do some fact-checking when you notice this happening. It may not eliminate whatever you're feeling, but it might slow a downward spiral or keep things from escalating further. If you're on a fact-checking mission, these questions can help you get in the habit of following your curiosity without judgment:

What's happening? Am I feeling emotionally triggered? Tempted to binge? Tempted to compensate for something I already ate?

_____

_____

What's the situation? Where am I, who am I with, and what are we doing? Notice the environment you're in and whether there's anything unusual about it that's triggering the emotions you're feeling.

_____

_____

Has this happened before? Can you think of a past event that could give you insight on how to respond in a helpful way?

_____

_____

What do I think this means? Have I blown this out of proportion, assumed a worst-case scenario, or interpreted it in a way that doesn't match the reality of the situation?

_____

_____

Does the way I feel match the situation? Is this emotion appropriate and helpful, or is it distracting? Can I move to a place where I can clearly think about my next move?

_____

_____

Am I judging myself for the way I feel about this situation? Are there other emotions at play that might impair my ability to make a decision or react in a helpful way?

_____

_____

Although it's not easy to remember to do it, practicing this skill can be done in a matter of seconds. If it's helpful, use your journal to keep track of your different responses to these questions and the outcomes. Over time, you'll be more adept at recognizing the facts of a situation and identifying your emotions toward it.

WHAT AM I REALLY FEELING?

It's entirely possible to understand the concepts and principles of intuitive eating and still struggle to see how they can help you. Humans are emotional and irrational at times, yet you can use curious questioning to get down to the root of what you're feeling.

This is a top-down approach that starts with a surface-level thought or emotion. By continuing to ask, *"Why does this matter to me?"* or *"What might happen?"* you may eventually arrive at a core belief. Once you've discovered a core belief, you can determine whether it's true and worth keeping or false and should be dismantled.

For this exercise, talk to yourself out loud. Practice in a manner that lets you focus on moving from one thought to another. Start with a feeling or emotion, and continue asking "why?" or "what?" until you reach a conclusion that reflects what you're really feeling.

Here is an example of a conversation you might have with yourself. See if you can relate to the **self-limiting thoughts**, in bold:

I'll never overcome my emotional eating.

"Why does that matter to me?"

Because I don't want to keep feeling out of control around food. **I'm addicted to food**.

"Why does that matter to me?"

Because it's distracting and I don't like how it keeps me from enjoying my food or the situation.

"What might happen if I keep doing it?"

I'll keep feeling tempted to restrict or diet, and my relationship with food will get worse.

"Why does that matter to me?"

Because I keep failing at sticking to diets; **I never succeed**.

"Why does that matter to me?"

I don't want to think of myself as a failure (a core belief that reflects what I'm really feeling).

Here's one more example:

I'm angry at myself for not exercising today.

"Why does that matter to me?"

It's important to work out. I don't want to lose fitness or gain weight.

"What would happen if I did?"

I'd end up right back where I started. **I'll ruin my health**.

"Why does that matter to me?"

I want to be healthy. I want to feel good.

"What would happen if you weren't healthy?"

I'm afraid I'll get sick or die sooner, and that makes me feel stressed and anxious (core belief that reflects what I'm really feeling).

This exercise isn't meant to offer an immediate solution; our fears and anxieties are often far too complex and nuanced to be mitigated by a step-by-step process. However, could you imagine living with a different perspective? Can you recognize the irrational aspects of your thoughts and beliefs and focus on the reality of what you have control over? Can you challenge your assumptions or look for evidence to the contrary?

SITTING WITH DIFFICULT EMOTIONS

Inviting tough emotions into your awareness can build resilience and greater connection to what you feel and experience in your body. It initially may sound like something you'd want to avoid, but that fear is often worse than the feeling itself. This simple meditation takes only a few minutes and can help you stick with your difficult emotions long enough to eventually move through them.

1. Start in a comfortable position, similar to when you tried the Body Scan Meditation previously (page 30). Close your eyes and focus on something that's difficult, whether it's a food you regret eating, the urge to revert to old habits, or a situation that triggers self-doubt. Acknowledge the desire to turn away from it and reach toward something familiar or comforting. You might envision yourself physically turning your back or reaching out your hands, but the way you visualize this may look different.

2. Now turn toward it. Take your time and, if needed, move your focus back to your breath. Start to envision the support you need to address the emotion. Compassion, strength, love, acceptance, security, kindness, non-judgment. Imagine yourself being covered with a blanket or cloud, or perhaps there is a figure that holds and supports you.

3. Come face to face with your difficult emotion, and offer yourself the reassurance that it will be alright. Silently say something kind and loving to yourself, and remind yourself that you're worthy of giving and receiving support. You are enough, and you are not alone. Repeat this as many times as needed until you begin to feel calmer and less judged.

Keep repeating this simple meditation until the emotion is more manageable. Each time, you may be less tense and compelled to turn away or more comfortable sitting with it for longer.

If you don't always have time to move through a full meditation, simply choose to observe your emotions, validate them, or label them so you can face them head-on later.

Taking Back Your Power

When is the last time you bought a big-ticket item? Maybe it was a home, a car, a major appliance. Chances are, you did a fair amount of research beforehand. You read reviews online, imagined your life after making that purchase, and asked for recommendations from people you trust. And with that information in hand, you were confident when you closed the deal.

In much the same way, it can be incredibly empowering to be so informed and aware of how you're feeling and why. Just like when you're doing the research before a big purchase, you're in a state of exploration or neutral observation. It's like the fact-finding mission where you recognize new information as one more piece of the puzzle that you're piecing together before you take action.

While you likely don't make big purchases on a regular basis, you do have opportunities to reclaim your power in smaller ways every day. This is where some of the nuance of intuitive eating comes into play—by approaching habits or activities from a place of self-care, without the intent of controlling your body or limiting food.

SHIFTING YOUR MIND-SET: WHAT'S THE INTENT?

By now, it should be clear that the point of intuitive eating isn't to change your body or revert to harmful behaviors. So what *is* the point? As mentioned earlier, being able to voice your needs and feel empowered to act on them is an essential piece of self-care because it's a means of providing what you know your body needs. But you may be wondering: Is this still a version of dieting?

For example, meal planning and prepping might look the same from the outside, but the intent and mind-set that's driving it can be much, much different. With dieting, meal plans are often restrictive or non-negotiable. They imply that you're succeeding if you are following their plan, and that you're failing if you deviate from it. Dieting leaves little room for flexibility. You eventually want to rebel against the rigidity of the rules and, as a result, become resentful, unhappy, or frustrated.

The food itself isn't the problem; it's the rules and restrictions around it. With intuitive eating, meal planning and prepping takes on a whole new meaning. Using a mind-set of self-care, you can introduce some flexible structure to the way you approach food. Perhaps one week you won't be able to cook meals as you normally would because it's stressful. You're sensitive to your budget, so you don't want to dine out, or you've made the connection that restaurant meals close to bedtime keep you awake at night. You decide to prepare a few things that can be thrown together quickly, but you remind yourself that if you decide to do something different for dinner, there's no judgment or shame. Meal planning and prepping is a means to minimize stress or chaos while providing something that makes you feel better.

JOURNAL: *What other scenarios can you think of where you can shift your mind-set from dieting to self-care?*

There's simply no way for any external food rule or diet to account for all of those things: They change on a daily—sometimes hourly—basis. With time and practice, it'll become less and less enticing to outsource your decisions about food to anyone but yourself. And that is where you can really take back your power from dieting and diet culture.

 ## PRESS PAUSE

Despite your best efforts to avoid or limit exposure to it, diet culture is everywhere. There will always be messages vying for your attention, trying to persuade you to come back to what you know. If you find yourself imagining what it would be like to try the latest diet trend, change the shape or size of your body, or let go of intuitive eating, there was likely something in your environment or thoughts that triggered that response. Instead of pressing pause on the work you're doing to heal your relationship with food, try pressing pause on the trigger itself. This exercise is easily done without a written response, but if it's helpful to you, it can also be recorded in your journal.

1. Start by recognizing the trigger. This may prove difficult if you aren't sure what the original trigger was, but try to identify where you were, what you were doing, or who you were with when those restrictive dieting thoughts popped up. Reflect on the physical sensations you felt (racing heart, flushed cheeks, tight chest, knot in your stomach), and make note of the emotions that came along with them (anger, frustration, annoyance, resentment).

2. Mentally say "pause" or "stop." You might visualize yourself shutting a door or literally pressing the pause button on a remote.

3. Bring your focus back to your breath, and take a few moments to ground yourself. Reorient to the present, especially if the trigger you're thinking of happened in the past.

4. Take on the role of an observer. Remind yourself that you don't have to rush into saying or doing anything. Notice your thoughts, and consider repeating some of the other exercises from this chapter.

5. When you're ready, press play and prepare to mindfully move on from these triggered thoughts and feelings that you experienced.

This might sound like a time-consuming process. But in reality, taking just a few seconds to pause, reflect, and observe can make a big difference in whatever actions you take next. Naming and observing your emotions may not influence your actions immediately; it can take a while to build resilience to your triggers and stop harshly judging your thoughts or feelings. At the very least, you'll be that much more aware for the next time the same trigger occurs.

Takeaways

- The mind-body connection is powerful and can have a big impact on health. Connecting with your emotions and understanding what they mean is a critical piece of creating well-being.

- Food can't fix your feelings, because there's nothing wrong with them. Emotions are important messages that can help you, regardless of how you might want to avoid them.

- Emotional eating is not inherently problematic; however, if you find that eating is your only coping mechanism, you may have the opportunity to find other coping skills that will support you in sitting with your emotions.

CHAPTER FIVE

Healthy FOOD, Healthy CHOICES

ONE OF THE MOST WIDESPREAD MYTHS about intuitive eating is that it has nothing to do with nutrition. Let's clear the air about this: Intuitive eating is based on nutrition science, evidence-based practice, and patient-centered care. It's about more than nutrition because a fixation on calories, fat, and protein alone (or the "food as fuel" mentality) fails to consider all the other ways food serves you beyond nourishment. Until you feel confident and empowered around *all* foods, restricting and avoiding foods will only continue the vicious cycle of the dieting mentality.

The Nutrition Foundation

Simply put: Food and nutrition play an important role in your life, but they need to keep their place as one, and only one, role. If you only paid attention to external cues like the media, recommendations from others, or the habits learned from past dieting attempts, it would be easy to assume that nutrition needs to be a top priority. However, these overarching recommendations do little (if anything) to factor in your unique needs. Not only that, but nutrition guidelines change and evolve over time in light of new evidence.

So can your habits and behaviors around food. The new evidence in your case is the reconnection you're working to develop with your hunger and fullness cues, food preferences, and how foods make you feel physically and emotionally.

There are times when avoiding or limiting a food is necessary. This might include foods you are allergic to or cannot tolerate, foods that don't align with your religious or ethical beliefs, or foods that leave you feeling less than your best. There is no rule that says all foods must fit everyone's needs. Over time, your body will begin to direct you toward foods that support health, and you will crave once-forbidden ones less and less.

WHAT IS YOUR INTENT BEHIND THIS CHOICE?

When dieting, nutrition is a big motivation. The goal may be to limit calories, get enough of a particular nutrient, or otherwise optimize health, but it can be confusing to try to differentiate between a dieting behavior and something that promotes self-care and well-being. There's an enormous amount of gray area in these situations, and if you're grappling with this, it may be a good time to start working with a registered dietitian who has experience with intuitive eating or a therapist who can help you navigate those waters.

In chapter 4 (page 57), you thought about ways to shift your mind-set away from dieting. Here are a few examples where your behaviors might look nearly identical but have an entirely different intent based on whether it's rooted in a restrictive dieting mentality or a flexible non-diet approach.

- Planning your meals because it reduces stress and helps you plan your grocery shopping—and not because you feel the need to stick to a meal plan or follow food rules.
- Eating single-serving packs because it's easier to stow packaged snacks in your purse or bag when you're on the go—and not because you feel out of control around a large amount of that food.
- Structuring or planning your movement because it's the most convenient time of day, you prioritize it as a stress outlet, you plan to attend a certain class you like, or you participate with someone else—and not because you feel the need to plan ahead to compensate for what you eat.
- Portioning foods because it's convenient to plan ahead or it helps you save money—and not because you're worried about eating too much.
- Declining a social invitation because you need time alone to relax or simply don't want to go—and not because you're anxious about what you'll eat or how you look.
- Reading about nutrition or health because you're curious to learn more and understand your body better—and not because you plan on trying something extreme to manipulate your body size.

If you're working through these nuanced situations on your own, ask yourself about the intent behind your choices for food or movement. Which actions are motivated by fear or discomfort? Those may be the areas where you focus efforts to ditch the dieting mentality. It can also be great insight into the progress you've made toward healing your relationship with food, movement, and your body.

BACK TO BASICS WITH NUTRITION

You may not want to reintroduce nutrition considerations too early; if you're still struggling with a diet mentality or holding out for weight loss, you may not be ready for this step. If that's the case, revisit the previous chapters and other resources (listed in the back of this book on page 112) before continuing with the rest of this chapter.

Keep in mind:

* The foods and meals you choose to eat should have adequate energy to sustain your body. You may need to consume more of the nutrient-dense foods you enjoy in order to get enough nutrition or feel your best (or include them more often when you have the opportunity to do so).

* Going longer than four to five hours without eating can disrupt blood sugar balance (when you're awake). This might sound like a long time or not very long at all depending on how often you eat now. If you don't normally notice your appetite, aiming to eat every few hours can be a good place to start until you are able to recalibrate your body's sensation of hunger and recognize it before you end up completely ravenous.

* Plan the foods you'll prepare according to your energy levels. If you know you'll feel drained and exhausted by the end of the day, include some convenience options. When you're more energized in the morning or on your days off, you can break out the cutting boards and skillets and make a more elaborate meal.

* If you're planning ahead for the week (or even just a few days), plan for three meals and a couple of snacks as a starting point. Just because you plan for them doesn't mean you must eat them, but you've given yourself the option.

* Including carbohydrates, protein, fat, and fiber can help you feel more satisfied and fuller from the foods you eat, as can staying well-hydrated. Notice whether you feel less energized or satisfied when a meal is missing one of these components.

When you learn to rely on your internal cues for what, when, and how to eat, nutrition suddenly simplifies. Just remember that no single meal or day of eating is going to make or break your health. You aren't doing yourself a disservice by allowing yourself to make mistakes or fumble through the process of becoming an intuitive eater.

The human body is efficient and resilient, and the work you're doing now will serve your health for years to come. It's okay to question whether intuitive eating is really going to benefit you. But if you trust the process and make peace with food, you'll see health benefits beyond the physical. Your mental and emotional health will also improve. In the long run, your overall health and well-being will benefit much more from having a peaceful, calm relationship with food and your body than it will by following the "perfect diet" (which does not exist).

Good Food/Bad Food

Intuitive eating strives to break down the moral value of food. It is impartial to labels. There is truly no right or wrong choice; it usually comes down to asking, "What is the best choice I can make for myself in this situation, based on what I know and what I have access to?"

Each person is unique, and, therefore, their relationship to food will be completely different. A single ingredient or food is enormously complex, and there are many considerations that must be factored in before eating it. For example, let's use spinach:

* Is it still a healthy choice if it's under an active recall for a foodborne illness?
* Is it still a good choice if it was harvested using the labor of underpaid or oppressed farm workers?
* Is it still a conscious choice if it's something you won't consume this week and will, therefore, be wasted?
* Is it still the right choice if you don't enjoy the taste or texture of it?
* Is it still a smart choice if it's beyond your budget and you must sacrifice something else to be able to purchase it?
* Is it still a sustainable choice if it's out of season and must be shipped across thousands of miles to reach your grocery store?

With a food allergy or intolerance, it becomes even more puzzling. Something that's "healthy," such as peanuts or dairy, can be a perfectly acceptable choice for one person but cause severe (read: life-threatening) anaphylaxis in another. There's also the added complexity of past experiences with a certain food that can create aversions or triggers. You might like the idea of a particular dish, but if it left you with a nasty stomach bug, you might have a hard time overcoming that aversion. Likewise, if a food was especially triggering for you because of a past eating disorder, you may need additional support to add it back into your eating pattern.

MY MOST RECENT MEAL

In a typical diet setting, someone might ask you to reflect on your most recent meal and think about how the nutrition and energy in that meal compared to your body's needs or a nutrition guideline. You might calculate the calories, grams of macronutrients (carbohydrates, protein, and fat) to see if there were any missing vitamins or minerals.

However, nutrition is only one small piece of a meal. In this exercise, challenge yourself to reflect on your most recent meal and think beyond nutrition. Use the space that follows to list or draw what that meal looked like and what you got out of it.

_____

_____

- What did I eat? How long ago did I eat?

  _____

  _____

- How hungry was I then? How hungry am I now? (Refer back to the hunger chart on page 41.)

  _____

- Was that food satisfying? If not, what was I craving? (Which flavors, textures, temperature, etc. did I really want to be eating?)

  _____

  _____

  _____

- What did my body need then? (To not be hungry? To address an emotional craving? To be fully satisfied?)

  _____

  _____

- How did I feel? Was I relaxed and at ease, or was I stressed or distracted?

  _____

  _____

- Where was I while I was eating? (At home? In a restaurant? In my car? At my desk? etc.)

  _____

  _____

MY FORMULA FOR BALANCED MEALS AND SNACKS

It's time to start brainstorming the types of food you want and need to include in a personalized eating pattern. This chart represents balance between the macronutrients (carbs, fats, and proteins) in a healthy meal using a combination of these types of foods. They're listed in this order to reinforce balance; when you're not including foods from all four columns, make an effort to choose from the far left and right columns. For example, combining a lean protein with a healthy fat might leave you feeling sluggish unless you also include a complex carb, fruit, or vegetable. Likewise, if you have only a fruit, vegetable, and carbohydrate food without trying to add a lean protein or healthy fat, you might feel hungry again a short time after eating and need another snack. Add foods to the list according to your food preferences and tolerance based on the general category of nutrition they contain.

LEAN PROTEIN	HEALTHY FAT	WHOLE GRAIN OR COMPLEX CARB	FRUIT OR VEGETABLE OR BOTH
Examples: Hard-boiled egg, canned beans, Greek yogurt, tofu	**Examples:** Avocado, olive oil, serving of raw nuts, salmon	**Examples:** Quinoa, steel-cut oats, brown rice, sweet potato	**Examples:** Sliced apple, frozen berries, salad greens
_____	_____	_____	_____
_____	_____	_____	_____
_____	_____	_____	_____
_____	_____	_____	_____
_____	_____	_____	_____

NOTE: There will likely be overlap between columns. For example, a sweet potato may be considered both a complex carb and a vegetable. An avocado can be considered both a healthy fat and a fruit/vegetable. Lean proteins, especially those from fish and seafood, may also contribute healthy fat. Keep this in mind as you build your meals to provide energy, nourishment, flavor, and satisfaction.

MY FAVORITE TREATS

Let's talk "treats." These are foods you may not have allowed yourself in the past; maybe they were considered too unhealthy or made you feel out of control. But planning to include fun foods that aren't for the sole purpose of nourishing your body is one of the most important aspects of intuitive eating. It helps break the cycle of avoidance and restriction and removes a lot of the novelty and temptation from these foods.

Do you find that you tell yourself any of these things about a particular food or food group?

- Once I start eating a food, I won't/can't stop.
- I've tried it before, and it didn't work.
- I think I'm addicted to my forbidden foods.
- I don't trust myself around food.
- My friends and family will criticize my food choices.
- I will criticize my food choices.
- I don't deserve to eat these foods until I lose weight.
- Other: _____

_____

If you answered yes, you may want to seek some additional support as you reintroduce these foods in a way that feels safe. If you have a hard time building confidence around these choices, it can be a slippery slope back to restriction. In many cases, attempting to reintroduce some or all of these foods at the same time can contribute to this, so start with one at a time.

Remember to offer yourself compassion and grace, as well as patience. Some foods may be somewhat easier or simpler to reintroduce because your relationship with that food is not as contentious or anxiety-provoking as others. Some foods might take many attempts and a much longer span of time before you feel as neutral toward them as other foods.

MY SELF-CARE LANDSCAPE

Life is complex; you can't sort home, work, food, movement, and the like into neat slots. As you progress with intuitive eating, you will learn to take a step back and look at the overall landscape of your life. You'll begin to see what you need on a daily and overall basis. Eating doesn't happen in a vacuum. Think about your must-haves for self-care and ease. That is, what products, foods, tools, and support do you need to have at home, at the office, and elsewhere so you can consistently nourish your body and practice the habits that are most important to you? Here are a few ideas to get you started:

- Grab-and-go prepared foods, frozen meals, or cans of soup so you don't have to cook from scratch or eat out every day
- A reusable coffee mug or water bottle so you can stay hydrated or enjoy your favorite beverage away from home
- A spare set of clothes, yoga mat, or pair of shoes that you keep in your car or by the front door for the movement you enjoy
- A small journal to jot down thoughts and feelings on the go
- A cozy sweater or scarf to keep warm at the office
- Hand lotion, lip balm, or a favorite essential oil blend in your bag
- A video or social media post that reminds you why you committed to intuitive eating
- Kitchen tools and gadgets (like a Dutch oven for soups, good knives for food prep, or an air fryer because you like crunchy foods) to help you cook

In addition, your self-care landscape might need to include some options that are readily available for when you don't feel like cooking or need some time for yourself. It's still important to nourish and care for your body even if hunger signals are absent or subtle or you're feeling tired or stressed. Your mind and body deserve to be nourished regardless of what you have already eaten or done that day.

PREFERRED CARE

Consider these questions as you explore your self-care preferences. As you experiment with the options you come up with, you'll learn what works best for your life.

1. What are some meals that are easy to prepare or pick up, taste good, and can sustain my body for a few hours? *Example: frozen meals or shelf-stable meals that only need to be reheated, recipes you can prep ahead of time, restaurant foods that you can pick up on your drive home, carryout items from your grocery store's deli section, etc.*

   _____

   _____

   _____

2. If I am stressed or tired, a meal might feel overwhelming. What are a few snacks that are easy to prepare or pick up, taste good, and can sustain my body for a couple of hours? *Example: packaged items you can add to your shopping list, bulk items that you can portion on your own, premade or prepared snacks from your favorite store, a fast-food item from a place close to where you live/work, vending machine items if you have to stay on-site.*

   _____

   _____

   _____

3. If I have had a hard day, what brings me comfort and joy? How can I soothe myself and feel more at ease? *Example: a favorite magazine, a new book, a hot bath, a massage.*

   _____

   _____

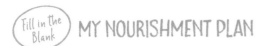

MY NOURISHMENT PLAN

This is your opportunity to take everything you've been thinking about and create a reference list to help you plan your meals and snacks. When planning food, it's sometimes simpler to account for the meals that are predictable or already taken care of. Maybe your weekday breakfast routine is simple, but you get more creative on weekends. Or perhaps your workplace provides meals or snacks, so you have less to plan for. And don't be afraid to factor in unknowns, too. Not having a plan can still be "planning"—this might happen if you're traveling or have a date night at a new restaurant.

Here's is a general template of a week's worth of eating. There is no right or wrong way to do it; you're the only one who can predict with any remote accuracy what you will need or want in the future. If this is just plain overwhelming or elicits any negative emotions, try doing one or two days at a time, or feel free to skip this exercise and come back to it when you're ready.

	MEAL 1	SNACK 1	MEAL 2	SNACK 2	MEAL 3	SNACK 3
Monday						
Tuesday						
Wednesday						
Thursday						
Friday						
Saturday						
Sunday						

NOTE: Just because you have a meal or snack planned does not mean you have to eat it. You've simply presented yourself with one option that can be changed depending on what the day brings. You might adjust the amount or opt for something else entirely. In the case of a snack, you could pass on eating if you're still feeling full and satisfied, or you might add additional snacks if hunger is more persistent or you're not satisfied yet. All of these scenarios will continue to teach you about your body and appetite, as well as how these planned foods impact you. Over time, you'll gain confidence based on how these past experiments have gone, and you'll be more efficient at working through this process.

MY FOOD SHOPPING PLAN

Grocery shopping can be an overwhelming experience—one that creates decision fatigue for some people. The grocery store may be a place where you've created food rules or felt stress in the past. In this exercise, you'll examine your habits, preferences, potential challenges, and obstacles. Once you've taken stock of how you like to shop, you'll plot out your next trip. Before you begin, know this: There is no right or wrong way to buy food. You are allowed to put whatever you want in your cart—no one (including you) gets to judge what you purchase.

What emotions come up when I think about shopping for food?

_____

_____

Where, when, and how often do I prefer to shop?

_____

_____

Is shopping something I enjoy or dread?

_____

_____

How do I feel about shopping with a list? Does it feel restrictive, or does it help me stay focused or save money?

_____

Do I want to buy the same foods every week, or do I crave new ingredients and variety?

_____

If I want variety, which new ingredients do I want to try?

_____

_____

When I get home, am I generally content with what I bought? Or do I feel like there's nothing to eat (or nothing I want to eat)?

_____

When I shop, do I consider my own needs and wants just as much as anyone else's (if applicable for families, partners, roommates, etc.)?

_____

After shopping for food, do I follow through with eating or cooking it? Or, do I struggle with food waste?

_____

What would it take for me to be more mindful when I shop, so I only buy food I know I will eat and cook?

_____

_____

Use the list of meals and food pairings you included in the previous two exercises and begin compiling a shopping list. In your phone or your journal, draft your list, either organized by store section or meals.

FINDING MINDFUL FORMS OF MOVEMENT

As you get more confident with checking in with your body and being more aware, you can begin to apply this mindful approach to movement. You may even land on an activity that you can consistently engage in, look forward to, and benefit from. Mindful movement prioritizes how you feel instead of the calorie-burning or body-toning effects. At the same time, it removes the comparison and competition that usually accompany exercise or workout programs.

Mindful exercise and movement can help you be more attuned to the subtle ways your body feels different from day to day. You'll start to notice when your heart rate increases, when you first start to settle into your breath, when you can push yourself, or when you need to back off. For this exercise, answer the following questions for each activity:

Walking or running on a treadmill

Does this activity sound fun or enjoyable to me right now? _____

Would I do this activity if I knew it wouldn't help me lose weight or change my body? _____

Is this an activity I'd like to try now or in the future? _____

What motivates me to do this activity? _____

Using an elliptical

Does this activity sound fun or enjoyable to me right now? _____

Would I do this activity if I knew it wouldn't help me lose weight or change my body? _____

Is this an activity I'd like to try now or in the future? _____

What motivates me to do this activity? _____

Attending a group fitness class

Does this activity sound fun or enjoyable to me right now? _____

Would I do this activity if I knew it wouldn't help me lose weight or change my body? _____

Is this an activity I'd like to try now or in the future? _____

What motivates me to do this activity? _____

Attending a yoga class

Does this activity sound fun or enjoyable to me right now? _____

Would I do this activity if I knew it wouldn't help me lose weight or change my body? _____

Is this an activity I'd like to try now or in the future? _____

What motivates me to do this activity? _____

Practicing yoga at home

Does this activity sound fun or enjoyable to me right now? _____

Would I do this activity if I knew it wouldn't help me lose weight or change my body? _____

Is this an activity I'd like to try now or in the future? _____

What motivates me to do this activity? _____

Using an online workout or video to exercise at home

Does this activity sound fun or enjoyable to me right now? _____

Would I do this activity if I knew it wouldn't help me lose weight or change my body? _____

Is this an activity I'd like to try now or in the future? _____

What motivates me to do this activity? _____

Walking outside on a sidewalk or trail

Does this activity sound fun or enjoyable to me right now? _____

Would I do this activity if I knew it wouldn't help me lose weight or change my body? _____

Is this an activity I'd like to try now or in the future? _____

What motivates me to do this activity? _____

Lifting weights or using weight machines

Does this activity sound fun or enjoyable to me right now? _____

Would I do this activity if I knew it wouldn't help me lose weight or change my body? _____

Is this an activity I'd like to try now or in the future? _____

What motivates me to do this activity? _____

Going to a boot camp or other high-intensity workout class

Does this activity sound fun or enjoyable to me right now? _____

Would I do this activity if I knew it wouldn't help me lose weight or change my body? _____

Is this an activity I'd like to try now or in the future? _____

What motivates me to do this activity? _____

Going to the playground with my kids or family

Does this activity sound fun or enjoyable to me right now? _____

Would I do this activity if I knew it wouldn't help me lose weight or change my body? _____

Is this an activity I'd like to try now or in the future? _____

What motivates me to do this activity? _____

Hiking

Does this activity sound fun or enjoyable to me right now? _____

Would I do this activity if I knew it wouldn't help me lose weight or change my body? _____

Is this an activity I'd like to try now or in the future? _____

What motivates me to do this activity? _____

Walking my dog or going to the dog park

Does this activity sound fun or enjoyable to me right now? _____

Would I do this activity if I knew it wouldn't help me lose weight or change my body? _____

Is this an activity I'd like to try now or in the future? _____

What motivates me to do this activity? _____

Playing a team sport or participating in a rec league

Does this activity sound fun or enjoyable to me right now? _____

Would I do this activity if I knew it wouldn't help me lose weight or change my body? _____

Is this an activity I'd like to try now or in the future? _____

What motivates me to do this activity? _____

Swimming

Does this activity sound fun or enjoyable to me right now? _____

Would I do this activity if I knew it wouldn't help me lose weight or change my body? _____

Is this an activity I'd like to try now or in the future? _____

What motivates me to do this activity? _____

Gently stretching while sitting, standing, or lying

Does this activity sound fun or enjoyable to me right now? _____

Would I do this activity if I knew it wouldn't help me lose weight or change my body? _____

Is this an activity I'd like to try now or in the future? _____

What motivates me to do this activity? _____

Working with a personal trainer

Does this activity sound fun or enjoyable to me right now? _____

Would I do this activity if I knew it wouldn't help me lose weight or change my body? _____

Is this an activity I'd like to try now or in the future? _____

What motivates me to do this activity? _____

Walking around a track

Does this activity sound fun or enjoyable to me right now? _____

Would I do this activity if I knew it wouldn't help me lose weight or change my body? _____

Is this an activity I'd like to try now or in the future? _____

What motivates me to do this activity? _____

Training for an event like a 5K or half-marathon

Does this activity sound fun or enjoyable to me right now? _____

Would I do this activity if I knew it wouldn't help me lose weight or change my body? _____

Is this an activity I'd like to try now or in the future? _____

What motivates me to do this activity? _____

Taking private lessons to learn a new sport or skill

Does this activity sound fun or enjoyable to me right now? _____

Would I do this activity if I knew it wouldn't help me lose weight or change my body? _____

Is this an activity I'd like to try now or in the future? _____

What motivates me to do this activity? _____

Another helpful question to ask as you reflect on your relationship with movement is, "When did it start to feel like exercising instead of doing something playful and fun?" These questions can help you differentiate between activities you enjoy that leave your body feeling energized and refreshed, versus activities you do because you hope they will result in weight loss or because you're accustomed to doing them out of habit or obligation.

You may still hope that mindful movement will change your body in some way. That's okay—it's normal. It's only an issue if it causes you to engage in movement that doesn't feel good or goes above and beyond what you can sustain for the long term.

WHY DO YOU CHOOSE TO MOVE?

There is no limit on the ways you can choose to move your body and experience the benefits of movement. Though you may struggle for a while to separate exercise and movement from their association with dieting or weight loss, there are many other reasons to move your body, either organically or in a more structured way.

Movement is part of everyday life, but so much focus is placed on the quantitative results. Fitbits, pedometers, and other activity trackers and apps provide external cues about your body, and they undermine your work to cultivate body trust and awareness of how you feel. Beyond that, no tracker is 100 percent accurate, and there's little science behind the "recommended" 10,000 steps a day. Getting caught up in the number of steps or calories or minutes you've tallied can blind you to what's really important. Does your body feel good when you move this way? Is there another form of movement you would enjoy more or be more likely to include in your routine?

Your effort and stamina will vary day to day, and fitness levels fluctuate over time. External cues are not reliable indicators of how much you should be moving or when. Just like you can relearn how to trust your body when it comes to eating, the same can be done with movement. Reflect on how you've moved your body recently. You move your body countless times a day in all kinds of ways, and most of them do not involve lacing up sneakers or performing intentional or repetitive exercises. You may have stretched in bed, then planted your feet on the floor and walked to the bathroom or kitchen. Perhaps you reached your arm overhead to scratch an itch on your back, or you walked from the parking lot to your office while chatting on the phone. Maybe you took your dog for a walk, played hide-and-seek with your kids, or practiced yoga to find peace and physical relief. Those are all intuitive reasons to move your body without trying to alter it.

For this exercise, revisit the list of different activities, sports, and styles of movement that bring you joy (page 90).

HOW I CHOOSE TO MOVE

Over the next several weeks, take time to reflect about how, when, and where you're moving your body. You can list your activities or organize them in a chart like the one that follows. If you are taking a break from exercise or structured movement, you may skip this exercise or track the times you decided against moving.

HOW I MOVED	WHEN AND WHERE I MOVED	WHO I WAS WITH	HOW I FELT

Periodically, check back in to consider:

- Did I enjoy this type of activity enough to continue doing it indefinitely?
- What aspects of this activity did I enjoy the most? (Where I was doing it, how it made me feel before/during/after, who I did it with, etc.)
- Would I still engage in this type of movement even if I knew there was absolutely no possibility of it changing the way my body looked?
- Did any part of this activity feel obligatory?
- Are there aspects of diet culture that could be triggering if I keep participating? (Considering what a trainer/instructor says, the advertising or media you're exposed to, what you hear or see while participating, etc.)
- Would I feel anxious or stressed if I didn't do this activity on a regular basis? What would it mean to me if I skipped this next time? How would I feel if I took a break from this activity?
- Does this activity ever cause me pain or injuries?
- Does this activity feel more like a burden or chore to get through, or more like a fun game that I look forward to participating in?
- Am I using this activity to avoid addressing something else, or is it adding enjoyment to my lifestyle overall?
- Can I afford to maintain this activity? (Take finances, time, and energy into account.)

Depending on your responses, you may want to adjust your approach to movement and exercise in the same way you've done with food. Remember that there is no right or wrong way, and it's always up to you whether to prioritize any form of movement in the context of everything else that's important in your life. If you need to temporarily take a break from a certain activity, or even all activity, that's also a very appropriate decision to help you heal your relationship with your body and practice a form of self-care.

Takeaways

- Nutrition is key, but it's not the only thing that's important. It will take some time before you're ready to include nutrition in your food choices again because so much healing needs to take place first.

- If you're still struggling with fear of certain foods or confusion about nutrition, please reach out to a registered dietitian who has experience with intuitive eating and can guide you through these steps with your unique needs in mind.

- Some flexible structure in meal planning or grocery shopping will help you maintain the habits that support your lifestyle. Avoid letting this structure morph back into rigid or restrictive food rules.

- Shift your approach to be mindful and conscious of how movement makes your body feel (just as you've been practicing with food and eating). It may be necessary to eliminate structured exercise until you can create a more peaceful relationship with your body and exercise.

CHAPTER SIX

CHANGE
for *Life*

Your Path Forward

If you have reached this chapter, take a moment to celebrate the fact that you've made it this far. It isn't easy, but you're taking some monumental steps toward healing your relationship with food and your body in a way you likely never have before. If this is your first experience with intuitive eating, stay open to the possibilities of what's to come.

It is a practice. Unlike dieting, there is no destination where you earn your badge of completion. As frustrating as that may be for some, it's actually one of the greatest benefits of intuitive eating. It can fluidly adapt to suit your current situation, and it can continue to evolve as your lifestyle changes during different seasons of life.

Going forward, you may feel more informed and empowered; after all, you (and only you) are the expert of your body! This journey involves a process of unlearning diet culture and relearning all the diverse ways your body responds to food, movement, stress, and so much more. You've already taken the first steps to get reacquainted with your body, so even if you don't feel like an expert yet, you will surely get there with more time and patience.

If it feels overwhelming to place so much attention on food right now, remember there are other ways you can rebuild body trust and establish familiarity with your body and how to care for it:

* Looking at your relationship with exercise and movement
* Honing your self-care activities
* Practicing mindfulness, not just while you're eating
* Having the tools to manage stress
* Taking care of your relationships

* _____

Intuitive eating goes far beyond "eat when you're hungry, stop when you're full." As you've seen throughout the other chapters, there are components of mindfulness, meditation, self-care, movement, and more. The common theme in all of them is to become less judgmental about your choices. This is especially helpful for challenges like cravings or emotional eating, which will inevitably come up. Intuitive eating helps you be more attuned to what your body needs and the way it communicates. As a result, you're more skillful and confident in giving it exactly what it needs.

And what exactly does your body really need? It usually isn't an expensive supplement. It might not even be eliminating foods from your eating pattern. It might just involve a little TLC in the form of discovering what makes you and your body feel its best and committing to that. So even if you don't have a current health concern or a desire to change your health, intuitive eating can benefit everyone. You may learn that you still need some support with fine-tuning your approach to your optimal version of health, but it is possible to do so without returning to restrictive dieting methods or extreme measures. However, if you've made it to the end of this workbook and still experience things like GI discomfort, stress, anxiety that seems unmanageable, confusion around movement, or you simply have more questions about your next steps, consider reaching out for more individualized support from a registered dietitian or therapist who has experience with intuitive eating.

LETTING GO OF WHAT NO LONGER SERVES YOU

You cannot move forward while looking backward. To embrace intuitive eating, you must let go of the hope that the next diet will solve all your problems. It's difficult to grieve the lost time, energy, and countless dollars spent in pursuit of thinness as health. It's normal and, in fact, quite common to experience feelings of anger or frustration about that. In addition, you may also be grieving an idea that you held in your mind for so long—perhaps a thinner version of yourself, or a version of yourself from the past, or the hope that you'd finally achieve something significant once you lost weight. In this writing reflection, you'll consider what you're now prepared to let go.

1. Are there aspects of dieting or past lifestyles that no longer serve you in the way they once did? Are there things you can remove from your life in order to clear more space for things that are now a higher priority?

   _____

   _____

   _____

   _____

2. On the flip side of that, it's possible that you still need more time to prepare to let these things go. Are there any ways that dieting and food rules are still serving you?

_____

_____

_____

3. If this is the case, which reflections or exercises from this workbook can help you continue your healing process?

_____

_____

No One's Perfect

Imperfection is part of what makes you human. You've probably learned that self-loathing or body hate hasn't yielded lasting changes. No wonder—it's really challenging to take good care of something you hate. Embracing your imperfections to the point of accepting and respecting them—even if it's still difficult to love them or feel positively toward them—is one way that self-love and compassion can encourage you to stick with this different approach.

In diet culture, there are seemingly endless food rules to keep track of, specific foods or ingredients to buy (and not buy), apps and tools to track all of it, coaches or gurus to report back to, and the list goes on and on. However, despite those challenges, it can still feel tempting to return to the familiarity and predictability of dieting even when you know diets will fail you again and again.

You might even be thinking, "What's the harm in returning to those habits one more time? Why can't this be the time it finally works and gets me where I hope to be?" That's part of the appeal of dieting, and it's an enormous challenge to let that go. It's human nature to want to feel supported and comfortable, even when things like food rules, extreme exercise, or body- and food-shaming messages make you incredibly uncomfortable.

HABIT BUILDER

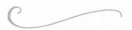

One essential aspect of self-care is creating boundaries for yourself and asking that they be respected. This is easier said than done because setting boundaries is something you do for yourself, not for others. It's a way of establishing what you will and won't tolerate and what you will and won't accept about the way you're treated. Suppressing emotions or deferring to others may seem unrelated to intuitive eating, but when you feel empowered and confident in other areas of life, you may find it easier to stay committed to your resolve to ditch diets for good.

Getting in the habit of speaking up for yourself and enforcing your boundaries isn't easy, but it is a skill you can improve over time. Start with a few simple phrases that you can practice until the words feel comfortable in your mouth. You may need to adjust these examples to fit your circumstances, but having something prepared ahead of time can make it much easier to get the words out when you need them.

When you want to decline being weighed at your doctor's office:

"I am not interested in weight loss, and I prefer to focus on other aspects of my health. I do not need to know my weight to be able to do that."

When you need to advocate for yourself in a health care setting:

"Can you please give me the same recommendations you would give to someone with a lower weight or BMI who got the same results?"

When you want to avoid a lecture about eating a certain way:

"I am not interested in changing how I eat. Can we please talk about something else?"

When you feel pressured to eat:

"Thank you, this looks great, but I'm actually feeling satisfied already."

When you need your friends/family/colleagues to stop engaging you in diet talk:

"I'm working on not talking about food or my body in a disrespectful way. Do you mind if we change the subject?"

When you feel doubtful about your abilities:

"I make choices to improve my overall well-being, not to control my weight. This thought that I'm having is temporary and untrue/unhelpful, and I can choose to treat my body well."

When you feel doubtful about intuitive eating:

"My weight, my health, and my worth are different and separate things. I can serve my health without worrying about my body size. I deserve the ability to trust my body and have a peaceful relationship with food."

When you are questioning what/how/when to eat:

"I have the right to enjoy food without guilt or compensation. I am still learning, and it's okay if I eat past my fullness. I have permission to skip the foods that don't satisfy me."

These are only a few examples of how practicing these statements can help you respect your boundaries when they are challenged. This list is by no means all-inclusive, so use your journal to continue practicing as needed.

And remember: Just because you ask for your boundaries to be respected once doesn't mean that you won't have to repeat yourself. It's okay—they're exposed to the same diet culture mentality that you've already moved away from. It can take some time and finesse to understand when others just need a gentle reminder and when they are genuinely trying to sabotage your efforts.

Be kind to yourself if you experience negative thoughts; nourishing your body and practicing self-care is a long-term project, and if you've been stuck in the cycle of dieting for years or decades, it won't be an overnight transformation. You'll have ups and downs, days that feel better than others, and perhaps even temporary breaks from focusing on this healing process. Don't beat yourself up if this happens; know and understand that becoming an intuitive eater is not a linear process. But rest assured in the fact that there's no such thing as "failing" at this. If you find yourself struggling, remember that this workbook and the resources within it can help you refocus back to the healing process you started and that there are many intuitive eating professionals who are available to support you along the way.

Hurdles and Wins

Though the challenges might seem significant, keep in mind how far you've already come. Simply picking up this workbook and getting started was a huge step! Consider some of the other ways you've already started to overcome some difficult things:

You've given up your safety net and committed to stepping into the unknown... but you decided you want to create a lifestyle free from rules and dieting, and find something you can sustain forever. Diets simplify food decisions by taking some of the thought out of it. You might have a meal plan or food rules or whatever other tools of dieting you used, but some of the decision-making was done for you. There's something to be said for that, especially in this busy, chaotic world. But you've cut yourself loose from that safety net and reclaimed your power in making your own decisions about your body and how you treat it. It can feel entirely overwhelming at times— intuitive eating sometimes feels like jumping into the unknown and trusting what you can't see or haven't been shown before.

You probably had to defend this decision... but you have the skills and exercises in this workbook to help you prepare a response so you can feel confident when the topic comes up. There are still many people who have never heard of intuitive eating. It's natural to question what you don't understand, and there are many, many misconceptions and misunderstandings about what intuitive eating is and is not. And people will likely try to draw comparisons to what they do understand, which is usually a diet. When you tell someone you're working on intuitive eating, he or she may assume you're in it for weight loss, not food freedom. Maybe you've stumbled over your words or had a hard time articulating what it is and why.

You might have to let go of relationships in order to enforce your boundaries . . . and the empowerment you gain from advocating for yourself can be a really incredible feeling, as difficult as it might be at the time. If this means you have to switch health care providers (if the option exists) to avoid continued lectures about weight loss or to disengage from an office friendship that's toxic to your healing process, so be it. Intuitive eating considers your physical, mental, and emotional health. So, if you're unwilling to discuss your body, your health, or your food choices with someone, you have to let them know. And if your boundaries are repeatedly violated, it might be time to speak up.

You had to build your armor against diet culture . . . and you might be amazed at how much space this creates for you to care about other things. Once you start to recognize diet culture, you'll see and hear it all around you. You can remove it from your life by unfollowing social media accounts that make you feel bad and tossing diet books and magazines.

You started to challenge your deepest thoughts and beliefs about food and health . . . this involves getting brave and standing up to diet culture. But if diets have left you frustrated, unhappy, or dissatisfied with food and your body, you're really taking a stand for yourself. Maybe you're still working through this, but perhaps you already started to see how many of these thoughts and beliefs are false. With time, you'll keep building the resilience to quickly identify them, reframe them, and move on without feeling compelled to act upon them.

You've battled through times when this made you feel anxious and stressed . . . but now you have chosen to spiral up and out of those feelings instead of starting the cycle all over again. Just because you've embraced intuitive eating and are trying to practice it for the most part doesn't mean you won't have moments when you feel like you're taking steps backward. Catching yourself reverting back to a thought or action rooted in that old mentality is part of the process.

Take some time now to consider your other victories, no matter how big or small!

MY BIGGEST VICTORIES SO FAR

What are my biggest or most significant wins so far? What is something I overcame that initially seemed daunting (if not impossible)?

_____

_____

What are some of the small things that now feel like habits? What do I notice myself doing?

_____

_____

Is there anything I've completely embodied so far? What are some of the things I do now that truly feel intuitive or simple?

_____

_____

MY BIGGEST CHALLENGES SO FAR

What continues to challenge me? Is there anything that still feels especially daunting or frustrating?

_____

_____

What makes me feel frustrated? Does it have to do with the time I need to invest? My environment? A lack of support? Distractions?

_____

_____

How can I address these barriers and stay true to what I know are the right choices for my body?

_____

_____

Finding What Works for You

As you near the end of the workbook, it's time to start putting together a vision of what you need to keep going. Much change occurs each day, so you'll want to have a flexible plan that can provide enough structure to help you stay accountable without becoming rigid or restrictive. See how often you can use a "for the most part" approach to the habits or goals you set for yourself.

If you can "for the most part" . . .

* eat a wide variety of foods, including those that provide the nutrition your body needs
* practice self-care in a way that serves you well and fits into your lifestyle
* resist the urge to judge your thoughts or actions
* set boundaries against messages of diet culture that don't serve you
* take care of your relationships so you have a solid support system behind you
* engage in some form of movement that feels good for your body
* avoid risky health behaviors, such as skipping preventative health screenings, neglecting mental or emotional health, and abusing drugs or alcohol

Use these ideas to create a template for what you'd like your days to look like. You might consider it a version of living your best life, whatever that looks like for you. You may even come up with multiple versions of it—templates for work days and rest days, weekdays and weekends, days spent traveling and at home—and one that can shift with the seasons.

	I NEED TO . . .	I WANT TO . . .	I WANT TO FEEL . . .	I WILL CHOOSE . . .
Food				
Movement				
Relationships				
Self-Care				
Personal or Professional Growth				
Fun and Pleasure				

For all the knowledge and understanding that exists for nutrition and health, there isn't a great deal of individualization. Rigidity and stress around food can contradict any health benefit that may come from the most optimal way of eating. Good nutrition will only help you if it doesn't come at the expense of other things that promote health and happiness.

It is your birthright to be able to trust your body. To have a peaceful and calm relationship with food. To have permission to care for yourself in whatever way you see fit. You have the right to be autonomous in your body and live by the code you determine for yourself, not the strict rules of dieting.

Remember: Bodies are not meant to stay the same. And you are not meant to stay the same.

This season of change and growth can be overwhelming and scary, but on the other side is the food freedom and body liberation you've been craving. Stick with it. I'm rooting for you.

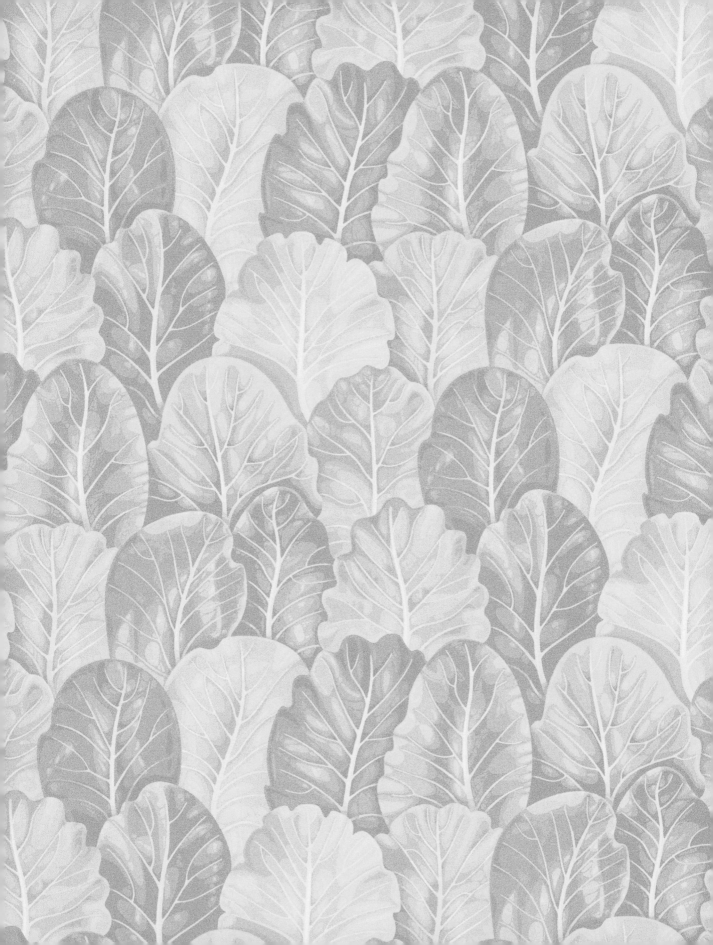

RESOURCES

These books, podcasts, and websites can offer additional support and information about intuitive eating, mindful approaches to food, and healing your relationship with your body.

Intuitive Eating (3rd Edition) and *The Intuitive Eating Workbook* (Evelyn Tribole and Elyse Resch): These books are essential reading for anyone curious about a non-diet approach. The third edition is updated with new information as well as a current list of studies that support intuitive eating. The companion workbook is a helpful tool for working through each of the ten Principles of Intuitive Eating with reflections, writing prompts, and other self-guided exercises. The online resources include a list of Certified Intuitive Eating Counselors who can help anyone get connected with an expert in their area.

Health At Every Size and Body Respect (Dr. Linda Bacon and Dr. Lucy Aphramor): These books introduce the evidence behind Health At Every Size® (HAES®) and debunks the myths and misconceptions around weight and health.

Body Kindness book and podcast (Rebecca Scritchfield): This practical resource helps readers create a happier, healthier life by shifting the focus from weight loss to well-being. Author Rebecca Scritchfield also hosts the *Body Kindness Podcast*, available on iTunes.

Food Psych Podcast with Christy Harrison: Dietitian and certified intuitive eating counselor Christy Harrison has been helping people make peace with food since 2013. The podcast explores a wide variety of topics in a non-triggering way, in addition to connecting listeners to an active online community for support with intuitive eating and Health At Every Size® (HAES®).

Love Food Podcast with Julie Duffy Dillon: Host Julie Duffy Dillon is a registered dietitian and food behavior expert. She explores topics such as emotional eating, orthorexia, women's health and fertility, and mindful eating. She also hosts a capsule podcast specific to PCOS called *PCOS and Food Peace*.

Unpacking Weight Science with Fiona Willer: This combination podcast and online community examines the flaws in weight science and challenges the widespread assumptions about weight, health, and nutrition. Audiences can also subscribe to the "Health Not Diets Digest" to receive updates about new research, hot topics, and top-rated articles.

Straight/Curve: This documentary tackles the issues, industries, and obstacles that contribute to body image issues among women and their lack of representation in media and the fashion industry.

Every Body Yoga (Jessamyn Stanley): Yogi, author, and activist Jessamyn Stanley created this body-positive, weight-inclusive yoga guide for practitioners of all abilities. Find easy-to-follow instructions for 50 yoga poses and 10 flow sequences, all photographed in a style that celebrates body acceptance and size diversity.

Association for Size Diversity and Health (ASDAH): This international nonprofit organization developed the Health At Every Size® (HAES®) Principles. The website provides ongoing opportunities for development, including educational resources, vetted referral opportunities, and an extensive network of like-minded advocates and professionals.

HAES Community (www.haescommunity.com): Find an extensive list of resources for Health At Every Size® (HAES®) as well as a location-specific registry of practitioners in various fields who have committed to a weight-inclusive approach by signing the HAES Pledge.

Beauty Redefined (www.beautyredefined.com): A nonprofit that promotes body image resilience through research-backed online education. The mission of Beauty Redefined is to expand the definition of positive body image and address the issues of objectification and unrealistic ideals of female bodies.

Underneath We Are Women (www.underneathiam.com): A multimedia project about body diversity. The photographs, social media and online community, and upcoming book promote a better understanding and appreciation for the diversity of women.

The Real Life RD (www.thereallife-rd.com): Robyn Nohling is dually licensed as a registered dietitian and nurse practitioner who specializes in a non-diet approach for women struggling with hormonal issues and period problems. Access online courses for healing hormones and regaining a healthy period as well as cultivating a healthy body image.

WellSeek Collective (www.wellseek.co): WellSeek is a digital media company on a mission to dispel myths and spread truth in the health and wellness world. Access curated collections of articles and resources for well-being of both body and mind.

National Eating Disorders Association (NEDA) (https://www.nationaleating disorders.org): The largest nonprofit organization dedicated to supporting individuals and families affected by eating disorders. NEDA also serves as a catalyst for prevention, cures, and access to quality care. It is the home of the NEDA Helpline to connect with information and support.

REFERENCES

Andrew, Rachel, Marika Tiggemann, and Levina Clark. "Predictors and Health-Related Outcomes of Positive Body Image in Adolescent Girls: A Prospective Study." *Developmental Psychology* 52, no. 3 (March 2016): 463-74. doi:10.1037/dev0000095.

Augustus-Horvath, Casey, and Tracy Tylka. "The Acceptance Model of Intuitive Eating: A Comparison of Women in Emerging Adulthood, Early Adulthood, and Middle Adulthood." *Journal of Counseling Psychology* 58, no. 1 (January 2011): 110-25. doi:10.1037/a0022129.

Bacon, Linda, and Lucy Aphramor. "Weight Science: Evaluating the Evidence for a Paradigm Shift." *Nutrition Journal* 10, no. 1 (January 2011). doi:10.1186/1475-2891-10-9. doi:10.1186/1475-2891-10-9.

Bruce, Lauren, and Lina Ricciardelli. "A Systematic Review of the Psychosocial Correlates of Intuitive Eating Among Adult Women." *Appetite* 96 (January 2016): 454-72. doi:10.1016/j.appet.2015.10.012.

Camilleri, Géraldine M., et al. "Intuitive Eating Is Inversely Associated with Body Weight Status in the General Population-Based NutriNet-Santé Study." *Obesity* 24, no. 5 (March 2016): 1154-61. doi: 10.1002/oby.21440.

Carbonneau, Elise, et al. "A Health at Every Size Intervention Improves Intuitive Eating and Diet Quality in Canadian Women." *Clinical Nutrition* 36, no. 3 (June 2017): 747-54. doi:10.1016/j.clnu.2016.06.008.

Christoph, Mary J., et al. "Nutrition Facts Use in Relation to Eating Behaviors and Healthy and Unhealthy Weight Control Behaviors." *Journal Nutrition Education Behavior* 50, no. 3 (March 2018): 267-274. doi: 10.1016/j.jneb.2017.11.001.

Clifford, Dawn, et al. "Impact of Non-Diet Approaches on Attitudes, Behaviors, and Health Outcomes: A Systematic Review." *Journal of Nutrition Education and Behavior* 47, no. 2 (March 2015): 143-55. doi:10.1016/j.jneb.2014.12.002.

Denny, Kara N., et al. "Intuitive Eating in Young Adults. Who is Doing It, and How is It Related to Disordered Eating Behaviors?" *Appetite* 60 (January 2013): 13–19. doi:10.1016/j.appet.2012.09.029.

Dollar, Emily, Margit Berman, and Anna M. Adachi-Mejia. "Do No Harm: Moving Beyond Weight Loss to Emphasize Physical Activity at Every Size." *Preventing Chronic Disease* 14, no. 34 (April 2017). doi:10.5888/pcd14.170006.

Duarte, Cristiana, et al. "What Makes Dietary Restraint Problematic? Development and Validation of the Inflexible Eating Questionnaire." *Appetite* 114 (July 2017): 146-54. doi:10.1016/j.appet.2017.03.034.

Dulloo, Abdul G., Jean Jacquet, and Jean-Pierre Montani. "How Dieting Makes Some Fatter: From a Perspective of Human Body Composition Auto-regulation." *Proceedings of the Nutrition Society* 71, no. 3 (April 2012): 379–89. doi:10.1017/S0029665112000225.

Gast, Julie, Hala Madanat, and Amy Campbell Nielson. "Are Men More Intuitive When It Comes to Eating and Physical Activity?" *American Journal of Mens Health* 6, no. 2 (March 2011): 164-71. doi:10.1177/1557988311428090.

Hawks, Steven, Hala Madanat, Jaylyn Hawks, and Ashley Harris. "The Relationship Between Intuitive Eating and Health Indicators Among College Women." *American Journal of Health Education* 36, no. 6 (December 2005): 331-6. doi:10.1017/S1368980013002139.

Herbert, Beate M., et al. "Intuitive Eating Is Associated with Interoceptive Sensitivity. Effects on Body Mass Index." *Appetite* 70 (November 2013): 22–30. doi:10.1016/j.appet.2013.06.082.

Homan, Kristin J., and Tracy L. Tylka. "Development and Exploration of the Gratitude Model of Body Appreciation in Women." *Body Image* 25 (June 2018): 14-22. doi:10.1016/j.bodyim.2018.01.008.

Humphrey, Lauren, Dawn Clifford, and Michelle Neyman Morris. "Health at Every Size College Course Reduces Dieting Behaviors and Improves Intuitive Eating, Body Esteem, and Anti-Fat Attitudes." *Journal of Nutrition Education and Behavior* 47, no. 4 (July 2015): 354-60. doi:10.1016/j.jnebA.2015.01.008.

Kelly, Allison C., and Elizabeth Stephen. "A Daily Diary Study of Self-Compassion, Body Image, and Eating Behavior in Female College Students." *Body Image* 17 (June 2016): 152-60. doi:10.1016/j.bodyim.2016.03.006.

Kelly, Allison C., Kathryn E. Miller, and Elizabeth Stephen. "The Benefits of Being Self-Compassionate on Days When Interactions with Body-Focused Others Are Frequent." *Body Image* 19 (October 2016): 195-203. doi: 10.1016/j.bodyim.2016.10.005.

Linardon, Jake, and Sarah Mitchell. "Rigid Dietary Control, Flexible Dietary Control, and Intuitive Eating: Evidence for Their Differential Relationship to Disordered Eating and Body Image Concerns." *Eating Behaviors* 26 (August 2017): 16-22.

Oswald, Alana, Janine Chapman, and Carlene Wilson. "Do Interoceptive Awareness and Interoceptive Responsiveness Mediate the Relationship Between Body Appreciation and Intuitive Eating in Young Women?" *Appetite* 109 (February 2017): 66-72. doi:10.1016/j.appet.2016.11.019.

Outland, Lauren, Hala Madanat, and Frank Rust. "Intuitive Eating for a Healthy Weight." *Primary Health Care* 23 no. 9 (November 2013): 22-8. doi:10.7748/phc2013.11.23.9.22.e754.

Pietiläinen, K.H., S.E. Saarni, J. Kaprio, and A. Rissanen. "Does Dieting Make You Fat? A Twin Study." *International Journal of Obesity* 36 no. 3 (March 2012): 456-64. doi: 10.1038/ijo.2011.160.

Sairanen, Essi, Asko Tolvanen, Leila Karhunen, Marjukka Kolehmainen, Elina Jarvela, Sanni Rantala, Katri Peuhkuri, Riitta Korpela, and Raimo Lappalainen. "Psychological Flexibility and Mindfulness Explain Intuitive Eating in Overweight Adults." *Behavior Modification.* 39 no. 4 (July 2015): 554-79. doi:10.1177/0145445515576402.

Sairanen, Essi, et al. "Psychological Flexibility Mediates Change in Intuitive Eating Regulation in Acceptance and Commitment Therapy Interventions." *Public Health Nutrition* 20 no. 9 (June 2017): 1681-91. doi:10.1017/S1368980017000441.

Sandoz, Emily, and Troy DuFrene. *Living with Your Body and Other Things You Hate: How to Let Go of Your Struggle with Body Image Using Acceptance and Commitment Therapy.* Oakland, California: New Harbinger Publications, 2014.

Schaefer, Julie T., and Amy B. Magnuson. "A Review of Interventions That Promote Eating by Internal Cues." *Journal of the Academy of Nutrition and Dietetics* 114 no. 5 (May 2014): 734-60. doi:10.1016/j.jand.2013.12.024.

Shouse, Sarah H., and Johanna Nilsson. "Self-Silencing, Emotional Awareness, and Eating Behaviors in College Women." *Psychology of Women Quarterly* 35 no. 3 (March 2011): 451-7. doi:10.1177/0361684310388785.

Steindl, Stanley R., Kiera Buchanan, Kenneth Goss, and Steven Allan. "Compassion Focused Therapy for Eating Disorders: A Qualitative Review and Recommendations for Further Applications." *Clinical Psychologist* 21 (2017): 62-73. doi:10.1111/cp.12126.

Tylka, Tracy L., "Development and Psychometric Evaluation of a Measure of Intuitive Eating." *Journal of Counseling Psychology* 53 no. 2 (April 2006): doi:10.1037/0022-0167.53.2.226.

Tylka, Tracy L., and Kristin Homan. "Exercise Motives and Positive Body Image in Physically Active College Women and Men: Exploring an Expanded Acceptance Model of Intuitive Eating." *Body Image* 15 (August 2015): 90-7. doi:10.1016/j.bodyim.2015.07.003.

Tylka, Tracy L., et al. "The Weight-Inclusive versus Weight-Normative Approach to Health: Evaluating the Evidence for Prioritizing Well-Being over Weight Loss." *Journal of Obesity* 2014 (2014): 983495. doi:10.1155/2014/983495.

Van Dyke, Nina, and Eric J. Drinkwater. "Relationships Between Intuitive Eating and Health Indicators: Literature Review." *Public Health Nutrition* 17 no. 8 (August 2014): 1757-66. doi:10.1017/S1368980013002139.

Warren, Janet M., Nicola Smith, and Margaret Ashwell. "A Structured Literature Review on the Role of Mindfulness, Mindful Eating and Intuitive Eating in Changing Eating Behaviours: Effectiveness and Associated Potential Mechanisms." *Nutrition Research Reviews* 30 no. 2 (December 2017): 272-83. doi:10.1017/S0954422417000154.

Wilson, Kelly G., and Emily K. Sandoz. "Mindfulness, Values, and the Therapeutic Relationship in Acceptance and Commitment Therapy." In *Mindfulness and the Therapeutic Relationship*, edited by Steven F. Hick and Thomas Bien, 89-106. New York City: The Guilford Press, 2008.

INDEX

A

Addiction, to food, 15
"Air food," 40
Awareness
    body, 52–55
    eating, 48, 50–51

B

Body
    awareness, 52–55
    -checking behaviors, 32–33
    ideal, 26
    -mind connection, 58–59, 75.
        See also Mindfulness
Body scan meditation, 30–31, 37
Boundary-setting, 103–104, 106

C

Challenges, 107–108
Change, 7
Checking in with yourself, 51
Comparisons, 32–33
Compassion, 34–36, 37, 84
Cravings, 62, 65–66, 69, 82, 100

D

Diets and dieting
    and community, 59
    culture of no, 21–22, 24, 77, 106
    feelings about food, 4–6
    food rules, 39–40, 73
    habits, 6–7
    hidden costs of, 27–29
    personal history, 24–25
    physical effects of, 22
    psychological effects of, 22
Difficult emotions, 71
Discipline, 15
Distracted eating, 44–46

E

Eating
    distracted, 44–46
    emotional, 14, 60–62, 63–65, 75
    environment, 50
    meals, 81–82
    and mindfulness, 47–48,
        50–51, 56
Eating disorders, 9, 19
Emotional eating, 14, 60–62,
    63–65, 75
Emotional health, 13
Emotional intelligence, 58
Emotions. *See* Feelings and
    emotions
Empowerment, 72–74
Exercise, 53–56, 78, 90–98
External cues, 18

F

Feelings and emotions, 59–60,
    67–68, 75
Financial health, 13
"Food Psych" (podcast), 24
Food(s)
    breaking the cycle of
        forbidden, 23
    feelings about, 4–6
    "as fuel" mentality, 77
    limiting, 77
    and mindfulness, 47–48,
        50–51, 56
    and moral values, 80
    and nutrition, 77–80, 98
    rules, 39–40, 72–73
    shopping plan, 88–89
Fullness, 41–44

G

Goals, 8–11, 108–109
Grocery shopping, 88–89

H

Habits, 16–18
    boundary-setting, 103–104
    emotional fact-checking,
        63–64
    listening to your body, 49
    "for the most part"
        approach, 108–110
Harrison, Christy, 24
Health, 2–3, 12–13
Healthy eating, myths vs.
    facts, 14–15
Hunger
    emotional, 58
    responding to, 29, 39–40
    spectrum, 41

I

Identity, 17
Imperfections, 102, 105
Inner critic, 28–29
Intention, 72–74, 78, 95–97
Internal cues, 18
Interoceptive awareness, 29–30
Intuitive eating
    benefits of, 2–3, 19, 100–101
    myth vs. fact, 14

J

Journaling, 7, 19, 34, 54, 73

L

Letting go, 101–102
Lifestyles, as diets, 15

M

Macronutrients, 83
Meal plans, 39, 48, 72–73, 78, 79, 87–88, 98
Meals
  balanced, 83
  eating, 50, 81–82
  nourishment plan, 87–88
Meditation
  body scan, 30–31, 37
  moving/walking, 55
  sitting with difficult emotions, 71
Mental health, 13, 58
Mindfulness
  and eating, 47–48, 50–51, 56
  movement, 52–55, 56, 78, 90–98
Mindless habits, 18
Movement, 53–55, 78, 90–98
Moving meditation, 55

N

Needs, 58–59
Nutrition, 77–80, 83, 98

P

Pausing, 73–74
Physical health, 12
Placeholder foods, 50–51
Portion-controlled foods, 40, 78
Preferences, 48

R

Relationships, healthy, 13
Repetition, 23
Replacement foods, 50–51
Restriction, 2, 6. *See also* Diets and dieting

S

Satisfaction, 48
Self-care, 72–74, 85–88, 103–104

Self-control, 15
Self-limiting thoughts, 69–70
Self-silencing, 58
Snacks, 83, 87–88
Spiritual health, 13
Suffering, 11
Support, for eating disorders, 9

T

Treats, 84
Triggers, 67–68, 73–74, 80

V

Values, 8–11, 58–59
Victories, 105–107
Vulnerability, 11

W

Walking meditation, 55
Weight loss, 14, 22

ABOUT THE AUTHOR

Cara Harbstreet, MS, RD, LD, is a Kansas City–based registered dietitian and nationally recognized nutrition expert specializing in intuitive eating and a non-diet approach. She is the owner of Street Smart Nutrition and the founder of Libre Connections. She also hosts the *You Can Eat With Us* podcast, which explores a wide variety of topics with guests who share their experiences with intuitive eating, joyful movement, and more. When she's not passionately advocating for a non-diet approach, you can find her enjoying a good book, exploring local running trails and new restaurants, or cooking up something delicious in the kitchen.

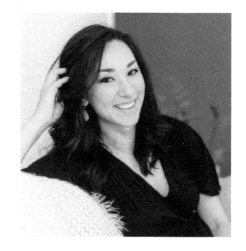